Anxiety Disorders

CURRENT CLINICAL PRACTICE

Neil S. Skolnik, MD, Series Editor

Anxiety Disorders
A Pocket Guide
for Primary Care

John R. Vanin, MD, DFAPA, and James D. Helsley, MD, FAAFP

*West Virginia University Student Health Service,
Robert C. Byrd Health Sciences Center, Morgantown, WV*

Foreword by
David M. Morgan, MD

*West Virginia University,
Morgantown, WV*

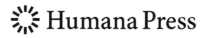 Humana Press

Due diligence has been taken by the publishers, editors, and authors of this book to assure the accuracy of the information published and to describe generally accepted practices. The contributors herein have carefully checked to ensure that the drug selections and dosages set forth in this text are accurate and in accord with the standards accepted at the time of publication. Notwithstanding, as new research, changes in government regulations, and knowledge from clinical experience relating to drug therapy and drug reactions constantly occurs, the reader is advised to check the product information provided by the manufacturer of each drug for any change in dosages or for additional warnings and contraindications. This is of utmost importance when the recommended drug herein is a new or infrequently used drug. It is the responsibility of the treating physician to determine dosages and treatment strategies for individual patients. Further it is the responsibility of the health care provider to ascertain the Food and Drug Administration status of each drug or device used in their clinical practice. The publisher, editors, and authors are not responsible for errors or omissions or for any consequences from the application of the information presented in this book and make no warranty, express or implied, with respect to the contents in this publication.

This publication is printed on acid-free paper. ∞

ANSI Z39.48-1984 (American Standards Institute) Permanence of Paper for Printed Library Materials.

Production Editor: Michele Seugling

Cover design by Nancy Fallatt

For additional copies, pricing for bulk purchases, and/or information about other Humana titles, contact Humana at the above address or at any of the following numbers: Tel.: 973-256-1699; Fax: 973-256-8341; E-mail: orders@humanapr.com; or visit our website at www.humanapress.com.

Photocopy Authorization Policy:

Printed in the United States of America. 10 9 8 7 6 5 4 3 2 1

978-1-59745-263-2 (e-book)

Library of Congress Control Number: 2007934680

Series Editor's Introduction

Anxiety disorders affect more than 40 million adults in the United States, or approximately 18% of the population[1]. Most of the treatment of anxiety disorders is prescribed by family doctors and internists. Untreated anxiety disorders lead to a great deal of unnecessary stress, fear, and uncertainty among a large number of patients and their families. Anxiety disorders encompass a number of different syndromes, including generalized anxiety disorder, panic disorder, obsessive-compulsive disorder, adjustment disorders, posttraumatic stress disorder, social anxiety disorder, and specific phobias.

In the primary care physicians office, anxiety often manifests as patients present with multiple somatic symptoms, and it takes a high level of suspicion, skill, kindness, and finesse to identify and address anxiety when patients are not aware that their symptoms stem from anxiety. Less often, patients come into the office seeking treatment with specific concerns about anxiety. In a recent survey, one-third of family physicians indicated a high degree of need for more continuing medical education about anxiety disorders and 78% indicated that they have a moderate or high need for continuing education about anxiety.

Anxiety Disorders, by Drs. John R. Vanin and James D. Helsley, fills an important void as a concise yet complete overview for primary care physicians of the most current thinking on the diagnosis and treatment of anxiety. The chapters are intelligently written with an emphasis on clinically relevant, evidence-based information that is useful in the treatment of our patients. There are chapters on psychopharmacology, psychotherapy, and each of the major anxiety disorders. Each chapter reviews the evidence supporting best practices in the treatment of each anxiety disorder so that the reader understands the full range of options available for effective care. It is a book that deserves to be on the shelf of all primary care physicians.

Neil S. Skolnik, MD

---

[1] U.S. Department of Health and Human Services, National Institutes of Health. National Institute of Mental Health – Anxiety Disorders. 2006 NIH Publication N. 06-3879

Foreword

As a practicing psychiatrist for nearly thirty years, I have known and worked with primary care practitioners who recognize and treat patients with mental disorders as well as any psychiatrist. I have also known primary care practitioners who have little interest in psychiatric issues as well as those who have considerable difficulty conceptualizing, much less verbalizing, treatment options for patients with these disorders. This is not meant to be a criticism. Practitioners who are not interested in mental health issues often have such a diverse and heavy general medical patient demand that excluding psychiatric disorders seems to be the least harmful option.

Although the exclusion of psychiatric disorders is completely understandable, it is impractical to disregard such a growing primary care practice issue. Psychiatric disorders affect all parts of the body and many aspects of everyday life functioning. Understanding how to better recognize, diagnose, and treat common mental disorders such as the anxiety disorders can actually help relieve patient demand and overall costs by correcting problems before they manifest themselves throughout all the possible avenues of care.

The ultimate goal of medical practice is to relieve suffering and make our diagnostic skills and treatment options the best available for our patients. This pocket guide is a tremendous addition for those who are interested in increasing their knowledge of mental health, particularly the recognition, diagnosis, and treatment of anxiety disorders. The details will expand the primary care practitioner's fund of knowledge and level of comfort regarding this large, yet elusive and complicated, segment of primary care. The material is thought provoking for practitioners who have had little or no experience in diagnosing and treating common anxiety disorders as well as for practitioners who are seasoned and regularly treat anxiety disorders and want to expand their knowledge base.

The quality of patient care will increase exponentially for clinicians who absorb the information that this book provides. This pocket guide is a real treat and long overdue!

David M. Morgan, MD

Preface

According to the National Comorbidity Survey Replication, the 12-month prevalence of adults in the United States with any mental disorder seen by a general medical professional is greater than 22% [1]. The level of disability among primary care patients with mental disorders is higher than many practitioners suspect, and can be greater than the disabilities from chronic general medical conditions such as hypertension, diabetes, arthritis, and back pain [2]. Anxiety disorders affect over one fourth of U.S. adults at some point during their lifetime [3]. In any 12-month period, nearly one fourth of patients with anxiety disorders are treated by a general medical professional [1], and these patients account for at least 10% of primary care visits [4].

This book is designed to help the primary care practitioner recognize, diagnose, and manage anxiety disorders in a busy clinical practice. The first several chapters give an overview of anxiety and the anxiety disorders, and provide the practitioner with practical information and techniques regarding the psychiatric evaluation and mental status examination in a primary care practice. Extremely effective modalities are available for the management of common mental disorders, including the anxiety disorders. The goal of treatment is not simply improvement but remission of symptoms and restoration of function. Some mental disorders, in fact, can be more effectively treated than hypertension or coronary heart disease [2]. This pocket guide includes helpful chapters on psychopharmacology, psychopharmacotherapy, and psychological treatment for the anxiety disorders.

Chapters relating to anxiety and the common anxiety disorders address adjustment disorder with anxiety, panic disorder, specific phobia, social phobia (social anxiety disorder), obsessive-compulsive disorder, posttraumatic stress disorder, and generalized anxiety disorder. Anxiety symptoms may occur due to general medical conditions, and this pocket guide contains a chapter dealing with common, potentially impairing conditions. Individuals with anxiety disorders may also suffer from coexisting mental disorders and are likely to have somatic or physical complaints. These complaints often mask the underlying problem and can lead to missed diagnoses, frustration, and high utilization of medical services [4]. The chapter on anxiety disorders and comorbidity reviews common coexisting mental disorders such as clinical depression and substance abuse. There are an estimated 78 million baby boomers in the U.S., and the oldest are now approaching retirement age [5]. Thus, there is a growing interest in geriatric anxiety disorders, and the identification and management of these disorders is vital. The chapter on geriatric anxiety disorders addresses the recognition, diagnosis, and management of anxiety disorders in the senior population and discusses several of the common medical disorders that may present with anxiety symptoms.

Timely consideration of anxiety disorders is important for appropriate management in a primary care practice. This pocket guide is intended to be a quick and handy resource for daily clinical practice as well as a practical source of information to augment other standard references and electronic media. Recommendations on collaboration and consultation with mental health professionals are provided, including resource information and a glossary of terms pertinent to the anxiety disorders.

The chapter authors have a combined clinical experience of over a century in the fields of mental health, primary care, education, and administrative areas. They have worked in multiple settings, including college health service, private general practice, academic inpatient and outpatient practice, military service, and community mental health centers. They are eager to share information about anxiety disorders from current research as well as from their experiences in the clinical trenches.

Becoming more comfortable with the diagnosis and treatment of the various anxiety disorders can be most rewarding for practitioners as well as for patients and their families. Appropriate management of anxiety disorders can make the difference between a patient feeling well with a good quality of life and living a life riddled with fear, tension, panic, avoidance, or somatic concerns. I hope that this pocket guide will provide information that is quick, interesting, practical, easy to read, and concise to help ease anxiety symptoms in your patients and, for that matter, in yourselves!

John R. Vanin, MD, DFAPA

References

1. Wang PS, Lane M, Olfson M, Pincus HA, Wells KB, Kessler RC. Twelve-month use of mental health services in the United States. Arch Gen Psychiatry 2005;62:629–640.
2. World Health Organization Guide to Mental and Neurological Health in Primary Care 2003–2004. http://www.mentalneurologicalprimarycare.org.
3. Kessler RC, Berglund P, Demler O, Jin R, Walters EE. Lifetime prevalence and age-of-onset distributions of DSM-IV disorders in the national comorbidity survey replication. Arch Gen Psychiatry 2005;62:593–602.
4. Feldman MD. Managing psychiatric disorders in primary care: 2. Anxiety. Hosp Pract 2000;35(7):77–84.
5. U.S. Census Bureau Public Information Bureau. http://www.census.gov/Press-Release/www/releases/archives/facts_for_features_special_edi.

Acknowledgments

Writing this pocket guide was an exciting, fulfilling, and challenging endeavor. We could not have accomplished this task without the support and guidance of many individuals. We both want to thank our lovely wives, Sandra and Vickie, for their love, support, and patience. They were always available for consultation and constantly helped to advance our writing, word processing, and editorial skills. We thank our children, family, friends, colleagues, and administrative staff for their constant encouragement and wonderful ideas. We both lost our fathers during the early phase of writing this book. These kind, wise men always taught us to do our best and pursue our dreams. We wish to dedicate this book to them and to our mothers who taught us to help others and share our knowledge.

A special thank you is extended to Richard Lansing, executive director for new project development, and the other editors and staff at Humana Press for their support, guidance, and positive attitudes during this long but most rewarding project. And finally, many thanks to the practitioners who read and use this pocket guide, for allowing us an opportunity to contribute some practical and scientific information for use in the daily care of their patients who suffer from the most common psychiatric disorders—the anxiety disorders.

J. R. Vanin and J. D. Helsley

Contents

Contributors

LESA J. FEATHER, PA-C • Physician Assistant, West Virginia University Student Health Service, Morgantown, West Virginia, USA

JAMES D. HELSLEY, MD, FAAFP • Associate Professor of Family Medicine/Behavioral Medicine and Psychiatry, Physician, West Virginia University Student Health Service, Morgantown, West Virginia, USA

KEVIN T. LARKIN, PHD • Professor, Department of Psychology, West Virginia University, Morgantown, West Virginia, USA

DAVID M. MORGAN, MD • Consulting Staff Psychiatrist, West Virginia University, Morgantown, West Virginia, USA

JOHN K. SPRAGGINS, MSW, LCSW • Director, Student Assistance Program, West Virginia University Student Health Service, Morgantown, West Virginia, USA

JOHN R. VANIN, MD, DFAPA • Professor of Behavioral Medicine and Psychiatry/Family Medicine, Director of Mental Health/Health Education, West Virginia University Student Health Service, Morgantown, West Virginia, USA

SANDRA K. VANIN, EDD • Commissioner, West Virginia Bureau of Senior Services, State Capitol, Charleston, West Virginia, USA

1
Overview of Anxiety and the Anxiety Disorders

John R. Vanin

Anxiety can be a confusing term because it can have several different meanings and apply to different experiences and behaviors. According to *Taber's Cyclopedic Medical Dictionary* [1], anxiety is a vague, uneasy feeling of discomfort or dread accompanied by an autonomic (self-controlling) response. Anxiety alerts individuals to changes, both within them and in the world around them, as part of an internal signal system [2].

Anxiety consists of a range of thoughts, feelings, and behaviors, and is influenced by biological, psychological, and genetic factors [3]. Anxiety is a normal but at times unpleasant emotion. The subjective experience of anxiety differs, but familiar presentations include symptoms such as apprehension, uneasiness, "butterflies in the stomach," anticipation, and dread. Objective behavioral manifestations include looking strained and tense, hypervigilance, shakiness, muscle tension, sweaty palms, rapid pulse, difficulty breathing, restlessness, and avoidance. Equivalent anxiety experiences may be described as nervousness, tension, worry, restlessness, irritability, agitation, and somatization [4]. Table 1.1 lists common subjective and objective symptoms and descriptors associated with various states of anxiety [2]. Although primary care practitioners are well aware of the many and varied presentations of anxiety symptoms and signs, they can present as true diagnostic dilemmas at times.

Individuals experience anxiety as a normal emotion at different times in their lives, and the source may be known, unknown, or nonspecific. Anxiety is a normal reaction to stress and can help one to cope. Anxiety involves anticipating future danger, and the response can actually help us to avoid potential danger—the "fight or flight" response. Triggers for the anxiety response include psychological threats, the unexpected, novelty, social/performance situations, cognitive mechanisms, and conditioned associative memories [4].

TABLE 1.1. Common descriptors and symptoms associated with anxiety

• Nausea	• Fatigue	• Tremulous
• Abdominal cramping	• Sleep problem	• Uneasy
• "Butterflies" in stomach	• Pupils dilated	• Worried
• Diarrhea	• Blurred vision	• Weakness
• Anorexia	• Preoccupied	• Wound up
• Vomiting	• Dread	• Flushing
• Urge to urinate	• Impending doom	• Pallor
• Dizziness	• Short of breath	• Headache
• Light-headedness	• Rapid breathing	• Tense
• Feeling faint	• Palpitations	• Terrified
• Jittery	• Racing heart	• Panicky
• Scared	• Dry mouth	• Phobic
• Anxious	• Lump in throat	• Restless
• Apprehensive	• Easily startled	• Shaky
• Keyed up	• Jumpy	• Sweating
• Stressed	• Chest pain/tightness/ discomfort	

Adapted from ref. [2].

Anxiety as a normal emotion can vary across the developmental stages of life. Young children may suffer from separation anxiety, whereas adolescents may doubt themselves and become very self-conscious [3]. A reasonable degree of anxiety can be adaptive. For example, anxiety as a normal emotion includes being nervous about going on a first date, studying harder for an important examination, feeling tense when starting a new job or when the boss is angry, or experiencing a rapid pulse and pounding heart when faced with a potentially dangerous situation. Anxiety can be experienced when things go right (e.g., a positive stressor such as getting a new, exciting job) as well as when things go wrong (e.g., a negative stressor such as losing one's job). Normal levels of anxiety essentially allow one to prepare for an action response of some type.

Anxiety can also refer to a symptom of an underlying general medical condition such as the nervousness and apprehension of hyperthyroidism, or a substance-induced symptom experienced from ingesting substances such as excessive caffeine or decongestants. Withdrawal from substances such as alcohol and other drugs can also cause anxiety symptoms. It is very important for the primary care practitioner to rule out underlying organic causes of anxiety because of the wide variety of physical complaints that incorporate anxiety. It is especially important to investigate possible organic causes in patients who initially present with anxiety in middle and late adulthood, have no apparent stressors or

TABLE 1.2. Examples of organic causes of anxiety symptoms

Medical disorders

- Angina
- Mitral valve prolapse
- Pulmonary embolism
- Congestive heart failure
- Cardiac arrhythmias
- Chronic obstructive pulmonary disease
- Asthma
- Hyperventilation
- Hyperthyroidism
- Hypoglycemia
- Pheochromocytoma
- Carcinoid syndrome

- Cushing's syndrome
- Meniere's disease
- Gastroesophageal reflux
- Irritable bowel syndrome
- Gastritis
- Premenstrual/menopausal symptoms
- Pain
- Seizure disorder
- Dementia
- Migraine
- Cerebral arteriosclerosis
- Akathisia (dopamine receptor antagonists, SSRIs)

Medications/substances

- Calcium channel blockers
- Theophylline/ bronchodilators
- Excessive thyroid hormone
- Hyperinsulinism
- Anticholinergics
- Steroids
- Substance intoxication/withdrawal

- Aspirin intolerance
- Excessive caffeine
- Stimulants/sympathomimetics
- Herbal supplements
- Monosodium glutamate
- Ephedra

Adapted from refs. [2] and [5].

family history of anxiety problems, or who are not responding to psychiatric intervention [5]. Examples of organic causes of anxiety are listed in Table 1.2 [2, 5]. The consideration of these secondary anxiety symptoms in the comprehensive medical evaluation of the patient is imperative.

Anxiety symptoms can become extreme, maladaptive, and disabling. Anxiety can affect an individual mentally, behaviorally, and physically. The normally helpful emotion of anxiety can be very disruptive and interfere with coping. Anxiety thus becomes pathological (a psychiatric disorder) when it is part of a group of symptoms and is associated with marked distress, impairment of functioning, and perhaps avoidance of people, places, and situations.

ANXIETY DISORDERS

Anxiety disorders are the most common psychiatric disorders in the world [5]. In the United States, over 28% of adults meet the criteria for an anxiety disorder in their lifetime [6].

The onset of an anxiety disorder is usually in childhood, adolescence, or young adulthood [5], and the median age of onset is 11 years [6]. Females are generally more likely than males to suffer from anxiety disorders. Anxiety disorders occur across all racial groups [5]. Anxiety disorders are serious medical illnesses that can be chronic and intense [7].

Unlike the relatively mild and short-lived anxiety that occurs with everyday stressful events, the anxiety disorders may become overwhelming problems and can grow progressively worse if not recognized and treated [7]. According to the National Comorbidity Survey Replication [8], of patients with anxiety disorders of 12 months' duration, general medical providers treated over 24% of them. The annual cost of anxiety disorders is in the billions of dollars, and more than half the costs are due to nonpsychiatric direct medical costs including undiagnosed, misdiagnosed, or inadequately treated disorders [5]. Improving the recognition, diagnosis, and treatment of anxiety disorders in primary care is vital to help alleviate the pain, suffering, and economic burden associated with these debilitating disorders that affect one in four U.S. adults.

The *Diagnostic and Statistical Manual of Mental Disorders*, 4th edition, text revision (DSM-IV-TR) lists the categories of anxiety disorders by signs and symptoms (Table 1.3) [9]. Each anxiety disorder has its own characteristic features, but the core symptom is the excessive experience of anxiety [4]. Practitioners may misunderstand anxiety disorders and not recognize their symptoms, especially since anxiety can manifest in different forms. Individuals may feel anxious and worry most of the time for no

TABLE 1.3. Categories of anxiety disorders

- Panic disorder (with/without agoraphobia)
- Agoraphobia without history of panic disorder
- Specific phobia
- Social phobia (social anxiety disorder)
- Obsessive-compulsive disorder
- Acute stress disorder
- Posttraumatic stress disorder
- Generalized anxiety disorder
- Anxiety disorder due to a generalized medical condition
- Substance-induced anxiety disorder
- Anxiety disorder not otherwise specified

Adapted from ref. [9].

apparent reason, feel fatigued, have difficulty concentrating, have uncomfortable feelings in social situations, have irrational fears or intrusive thoughts, exhibit avoidance behaviors, or suffer from periods of intense and terrifying feelings that can be immobilizing. Some patients misinterpret anxious feelings as depression. All the anxiety disorders may include some degree of situational anxiety symptoms [2]. Common, formal (primary) anxiety disorders include generalized anxiety disorder, panic disorder, obsessive-compulsive disorder, phobias (specific, social phobia [social anxiety disorder]), and posttraumatic stress disorder. Table 1.4 lists examples of different forms of anxiety with a brief description and a peak age period at onset [2, 3, 10].

It is important to distinguish the anxiety disorders from one another as well as from other psychiatric disorders. The focus of the anxiety and the specific cluster of symptoms help to distinguish among the different anxiety disorder categories [11]. A specific diagnosis may determine specific treatment decisions by the clinician. For example, it is imperative to start antidepressants in low doses and slowly titrate upward in a patient with generalized anxiety disorder and panic disorder to avoid or minimize jitteriness or exacerbation of the anxiety symptoms. Also, higher ultimate doses of antidepressants such as the selective serotonin reuptake inhibitors may be required for the treatment of obsessive-compulsive symptoms. Simple phobias are known generally not to be responsive to medications and require treatment with psychotherapy such as cognitive-behavior therapy.

Anxiety disorders often coexist with other anxiety disorders. Packaging the anxiety disorders into nice, neat categories is helpful, but the practitioner must keep in mind that real life presentations of

TABLE 1.4. Specific anxiety disorders, brief description, and peak periods of onset

Specific phobias: innate, conditioned, learned fears	Middle childhood
Social phobias: shyness, social discomfort	Middle adolescence
Panic disorder: panic attacks	Late adolescence
Generalized anxiety disorder: excessive worry about consequences	Young adulthood
Obsessive-compulsive disorder: repetitive thoughts, rituals, acts	Early adulthood
Posttraumatic stress disorder: anxiety from traumatic experiences (age of onset depends on precipitating event)	Childhood/later

Adapted from refs. [2], [3], and [10].

these disorders often do not appear in this manner. The comorbidity with other disorders such as depression, bipolar disorder, eating disorders, substance use disorders, and adult attention deficit disorder can complicate both the diagnosis and treatment of anxiety disorders. There is also an increased risk for suicidal behaviors with comorbid disorders [5].

BIOPSYCHOSOCIAL FACTORS

It is important to consider several factors when evaluating a patient for anxiety disorders. There is a complex interaction among these factors that includes genetics, psychological and life experiences, as well as brain chemistry. Although everyone has experienced stress and anxiety at one time or another, not everyone develops an anxiety disorder. Genetic variations may predispose an individual to anxiety disorders. The serotonin transporter gene variation is an example of a specific problem that may lead to low serotonin levels [3]. There are probably several genes involved in anxiety disorders. Family, twin, and adoption studies have shown heredity to be a factor regarding anxiety disorders. Heredity has been recognized since the late 19th century as an important factor in individuals with anxiety disorders [12]. Individuals who have a first-degree relative such as a parent or sibling with an anxiety disorder are at an increased risk for developing an anxiety disorder [3]. Researchers continue to pursue genetic linkage information and the identification of specific genes and areas of genes that may be associated with the vulnerability to anxiety disorders.

Psychological factors are also associated with anxiety disorder symptoms. Individuals prone to anxiety sensitivity may misinterpret bodily cues [10]. Common physiological symptoms may be misinterpreted as a significant or dangerous problem, and this may lead to fear and anxiety symptoms. Other psychological aspects common to anxiety disorders include the emotion of anxiety, associated cognitions related to the threat of harm, and behaviors related to preventing, avoiding, or escaping anticipated harm [11]. For example, an individual may suffer with panic attacks and misinterpret the increased heart rate, chest discomfort, and light-headedness as symptoms of a heart attack or a stroke. Concerns about having the next episode can lead to anticipatory anxiety and perhaps avoidance of a place or situation associated with an attack, where escape may be deemed as a difficult or impossible task.

Psychodynamic theories also remain as significant factors in the understanding of anxiety disorders [12]. Janet postulated that anxiety disorder symptoms resulted from an ego weakened by psychological trauma that led to a loss of emotional control [13]. Freud initially theorized the ego as being strong and resilient against trauma, and able to repress memories and their associated painful affect and transform them via psychodynamic defenses into psychoneurotic symptoms [13]. Later, Freud studied clinical anxiety and concluded that anxiety is physiological and remained outside the bounds of psychodynamic theory. A practitioner who is psychodynamically oriented views anxiety as a manifestation of an underlying psychological conflict that can be explored and resolved. The primary focus includes the patient's thoughts, feelings, fantasies, perceptions, and memories [13].

Temperament may also affect an individual's predisposition to anxiety disorders. Temperament is a combination of emotional reactivity as well as intellectual, ethical, and physical characteristics that remain fairly stable over time [1, 3]. Researchers have noted that some children are born with a temperamental bias called behavioral inhibition that manifests as increased physiological reactivity and anxiety in unfamiliar environments [10].

Environmental and social factors are involved in the development of anxiety disorders, including learned behaviors. Risk factors for the development of anxiety disorders in children include parental overprotection, excessive criticism, and lack of warmth [10]. Other environmental risk factors include social isolation, poverty, repeated personal losses, and exposure to violence [10].

UNDERSTANDING FEAR AND ANXIETY

To better understand anxiety, it is helpful to take a closer look at the fear response. Fear is a normal response to a threat, whereas anxiety is an unwarranted or inappropriate fear [4]. Anxiety and fear do not have to be learned. They are unconditioned, protective responses. The fear/anxiety response includes defensive behaviors, arousal of the autonomic system, increase in somatic reflexes, and activation of the hypothalamic-pituitary-adrenal axis [4].

Several parts of the brain are involved in fear and anxiety. Neurochemical studies and brain imaging techniques have improved the understanding of the complex network of interacting structures responsible for these emotions [7]. The cerebral cortex and the amygdala are two major brain areas involved in the perception of a threat. The cortex is the thinking or cognitive portion of the brain. The amygdala is an almond-shaped structure that serves as a communications center for the parts of the brain that process incoming sensory signals and interprets the information. It is involved in rapid, automatic responses that prepare the brain and body to deal with danger and the unexpected [3]. The fear response via the amygdala occurs before the cortical response, and so the response may be "automatic" without the individual having time to actually think about any action. The amygdala can register the presence of a threat, trigger a fear response or anxiety, and store emotional memories [7]. Various anxiety symptoms may occur including an increased startle response, hypervigilance, shortness of breath, and a facial expression of fear [4]. Increased output from the amygdala is common with the anxiety disorders.

The body's response to a threat also involves the activation of the hypothalamus, which serves as a command center for the hormonal and nervous system of the body [3]. Neurotransmitters are chemical messengers within the brain, and hormones carry messages throughout the body. The hypothalamus releases corticotropin-releasing factor (CRF) that triggers the release of adrenocorticotropic hormone (ACTH) from the pituitary gland. Adrenocorticotropic hormone stimulates the release of cortisol from the adrenal gland. This stress hormone is released into the bloodstream and has a regulatory effect on the brain, maintaining physiologic integrity. Cortisol is involved in complex negative feedback loops [14]. Excessive and sustained secretion of cortisol, however, can lead to adverse medical effects [14]. The adrenal medulla has direct communication with the brain by way of the sympathetic nervous system. The release of catecholamines prepares an individual for the "fight or flight" response by causing such responses as an increased heart rate and blood pressure, a diversion of blood from the internal organs to the muscles, increasing alertness, and increasing glucose to provide energy.

The hippocampus is a brain structure that processes traumatic stimuli and helps to encode the information into memories. Associated cues are stored in the hippocampus, and these may allow an individual to avoid stimuli that may trigger emotional trauma in the future [4]. Studies have shown that the hippocampus appears to be smaller in patients who have suffered severe stress such as combat or child abuse [7].

Cognitive control of anxiety occurs in the medial frontal cortex that is connected to the amygdala. This allows an individual rationally to evaluate a situation, regulate affect, control behavioral and interpersonal responses, and modulate autonomic and neuroendocrine function [3, 4]. If the stressors are particularly challenging, the lower centers such as the amygdala take over from the executive centers in the prefrontal cortex [4]. When a person suffers from an anxiety disorder, the response tends to be limited to the amygdala-mediated pathways, which can be pathological. Different parts of the amygdala may be activated with the different anxiety disorders and results in different manifestations of anxiety [3]. For example, individuals with panic attacks have a fear of dying. Free-floating anxiety is common with generalized anxiety disorder. Fear of embarrassment is a typical symptom with social anxiety disorder. Intrusive obsessions are common with obsessive-compulsive disorder. Emotional memory is common with posttraumatic stress disorder [4].

There are several other brain structures involved in fear and anxiety. These include the cingulate, basal ganglia, and striatum.

Life-threatening traumatic experiences can be etched into the amygdala. New favorable memories can decrease more threatening memories. However, new traumatic experiences or associations can trigger original, unfavorable experiences [4]. Anxiety tends to occur with limited patterns of thinking and behavior and is associated with circuits that are emotionally driven [4]. The fear response, therefore, can be automatic and lifesaving in situations of real danger. On the other hand, the anxiety response, as part of a learned fear response, may be an overreaction to a relatively benign situation that can be problematic and can perhaps be disabling. A core problem in anxiety disorders is a faulty connection between a stimulus and a response as well as a misinterpretation of an event's meaning [3].

ANXIETY: NEURONS AND NEUROCHEMISTRY

Several neurotransmitters (chemical messengers) in distinct areas of the brain have been demonstrated to play a role in the neurobiology of fear and anxiety [14]. Long-term dysregulation of these substances have effects on cortical and subcortical areas, and this appears to contribute to the development of anxiety disorders [14]. Research in animal physiology and human pharmacological studies have indicated that the familiar neurotransmitters γ-aminobutyric acid (GABA), norepinephrine, and serotonin are involved in anxiety disorders [15]. Other neurotransmitters and neuropeptides that interact and modulate fear and anxiety include CRF, neuropeptide Y, galanin, substance P, a variety of opioids, dopamine, glutamate, amino acid transmitters, and adrenal steroids such as cortisol [14–16]. Cholecystokinin (CCK), a neuropeptide found in the gastrointestinal (GI) tract and the brain, is the only circulating endogenous peptide that is known to be anxiogenic in humans [14, 15].

These neurochemicals, which work in various systems, play important adaptive roles in responding to stress, which include affecting energy stores, attention, vigilance, memory, planning, and cardiovascular function [14, 16]. Chronic activation, however, can be problematic. Clinically, several classes of medications are available that affect many of the neurotransmitters and are helpful in managing the primary anxiety disorders. These include the benzodiazepines, serotonin-1A agonists, and antidepressants affecting serotonin and norepinephrine [4].

HOW A NEURON WORKS

When a neuron (nerve cell) is activated, an electrical signal travels down the axon and releases a neurotransmitter. The neurotransmitter carries a chemical message across the synaptic cleft, attaches to a receptor on the receiving neuron, and transmits an excitatory or inhibitory message. Feedback mechanisms serve as regulators for the neurons sending the messages, and a reuptake transporter protein returns the neurotransmitter back across the synapse to the sending neuron after the job is completed. At times this complex system develops problems that manifest clinically as psychiatric disorders, including anxiety disorders. Problems with neurotransmission may include receptor hypersensitivity or hyposensitivity, deficient neurotransmitter release, and reuptake occurring too quickly [3].

As mentioned previously, anxiety occurs as a normal adaptive response to a threat and may be accompanied by increased autonomic (sympathetic and parasympathetic) activity [17]. The autonomic nervous system controls involuntary function of the internal organs and is involved in the fear response [3]. Abnormal anxiety with physiological activation has been shown to include somatic concerns. For example, studies have shown that a history of anxiety disorders is associated with an increased risk for coronary heart disease, including sudden cardiac death, compared to a history without anxiety problems [17].

SEROTONIN SYSTEM

The primary source of serotonin in the central nervous system (CNS) is the raphe nuclei of the brainstem. Serotonin has modulating effects on the locus ceruleus and its projections to the amygdala [4]. It is also associated with cognitive function in anxiety as well as regulating anxiety and impulsivity in suicidal behavior and other violence [4]. Low levels of serotonin are also associated with dysregulation of other neurotransmitters.

NOREPINEPHRINE (NORADRENERGIC) SYSTEM

The majority of the noradrenergic neurons are located in the locus ceruleus in the dorsal pons. Other areas of the brain that contain noradrenergic neurons include the limbic system (hypothalamus, hippocampus, and amygdala) as well as the cerebral cortex [14]. Autonomic arousal occurs with stimulation of the locus ceruleus, and the elevated norepinephrine levels are associated with somatic anxiety symptoms such as a rapid heart rate and increased blood pressure [4]. Chronic symptoms of increased noradrenergic function in patients with anxiety disorders include startle response, insomnia, and panic attacks [14]. Anxiety is associated with an increase in the norepinephrine metabolite 3-methoxy-4-hydroxy-phenylglycol (MHPG). There is a high concentration of GABA (inhibitory neurotransmitter) receptors on the noradrenergic cell bodies in the locus ceruleus [4].

γ-AMINOBUTYRIC ACID

γ-Aminobutyric acid is an inhibitory neurotransmitter in the CNS. It regulates or inhibits other neurotransmitters, such as serotonin, norepinephrine, and dopamine [4], and this neuromodulation affects arousal. There are both GABA-A and GABA-B receptors. γ-Aminobutyric acid exists only in the CNS.

TREATMENT OF ANXIETY DISORDERS

History of Treatment

Psychoanalysis and barbiturates were the primary treatment modalities until the mid-20th century. Psychoanalysis, although not empirically shown to be efficacious for the anxiety disorders, helps one to understand the roots of anxiety [18]. Pharmacologically, the barbiturates were widely used to treat anxiety. However, they have the potential for physical dependence and risk of misuse, including being dangerous in overdose. The benzodiazepines, which are partial agonists for the GABA-A receptors, were discovered in the 1960s. They are widely used to treat anxiety disorders. Researchers in the 1960s also found that the tricyclic antidepressant imipramine (Tofranil) reduced panic attack frequency [18, 19]. Since the 1980s, selective serotonin reuptake inhibitors (SSRIs), starting with fluoxetine (Prozac), have been utilized for the treatment of anxiety disorders.

Regarding the psychological therapies, cognitive-behavioral therapy has been empirically validated for anxiety disorders [18]. The overall efficacy of medications for the anxiety disorders is similar to the best psychological therapies, but there appears to be a longer-lasting therapeutic benefit with the psychological therapies [18]. For many patients, a combination of pharmacotherapy and psychotherapy seems to work best.

Primary Care Assessment

In the comprehensive evaluation, a primary care practitioner must always think about the categories of anxiety disorders, including patients with chronic general medical problems. The practitioner must also consider coexisting psychiatric disorders including depression, bipolar disorder, eating disorders, adult attention deficit hyperactivity disorder, and alcohol and other substance abuse. There is no substitute for spending a little extra time with the patient and listening carefully. Close observation and involvement of the patient in the discussion is very important in the evaluation of anxiety disorders. Education is vital to helping the patient understand and deal with the various ramifications of anxiety disorder symptoms. It is also not uncommon for anxious patients to question their diagnosis and demonstrate ambivalence and apprehension about their treatment. Patience and persistence is required of both the practitioner and the patient.

Anxiety becomes a clinical diagnosis when the symptoms become distressing and interferes with a patient's functioning. Anxiety disorders are commonly encountered in the primary care setting. Most patients with anxiety disorders have at least one serious general medical problem and a significantly higher probability for physical illness than those who do not suffer from anxiety disorders [20]. Anxiety disorders can affect all bodily systems including the gastrointestinal, respiratory, cardiovascular, endocrine, neurologic, and rheumatologic. Individuals with anxiety disorders also suffer from higher rates of allergies [20]. Many clinicians consider anxiety disorders as conditions that are brief and benign, but they can be truly chronic, serious, at times disabling conditions.

It is important to remember that diagnosing anxiety disorders is based on the direct clinical interview and the observation of objective manifestations of anxiety [21]. Self-report and clinician-administered checklists can be extremely valuable adjuncts in the assessment and follow-up of anxiety symptoms as well.

Treatment Modalities
Psychotherapy and medications are important treatment modalities for anxiety disorders. Both are effective for most anxiety disorders, and the choice depends on many factors including patient preference, practitioner preference, previous treatment, family history, availability, and cost. The efficacy of medication for anxiety disorders is similar to the best psychological therapies. There appears to be a longer-lasting therapeutic benefit with the psychological therapies [18]. For many patients, a combination of pharmacotherapy and psychotherapy is the best approach to treatment.

Psychotherapy

Cognitive behavior therapy (CBT) has been empirically validated for the treatment of anxiety disorders [18]. There are patients, however, who respond incompletely or not at all to CBT [10]. Psychotherapy alone may be helpful as a first-line form of treatment for patients with mild anxiety such as situational or adjustment problems. A brief course of a rapid-acting anxiolytic such as a benzodiazepine may also be helpful in these patients. Patients who have anxiety disorders and prefer to avoid the use of medications may also benefit from psychotherapy.

The cognitive component of CBT helps patients modify distorted or inaccurate thinking patterns. The behavioral component helps patients change their reactions to situations that induce anxiety symptoms. Behavioral components include exposure (confronting fear), response prevention (kept from performing behaviors), and relaxation, including deep-breathing exercises. The major aim of cognitive-behavioral and behavioral therapy is to eliminate beliefs and behaviors that maintain anxiety symptoms [7]. In particular, CBT attempts to increase cognitive control over the fear response [3]. The primary side effect of these forms of psychotherapy appears to be temporary discomfort due to increased anxiety levels [7].

Pharmacotherapy

The pharmacological treatment of most anxiety disorders includes the selective serotonin reuptake inhibitors (SSRIs), serotonin-norepinephrine reuptake inhibitors (SNRIs), benzodiazepines, and the nonbenzodiazepine 5-hydroxytryptamine (5-HT1A) receptor agonist buspirone (BuSpar). It is important to consider comorbidity when a practitioner selects a medication regimen to treat an anxiety disorder [22].

There are several medications approved by the U.S. Food and Drug Administration (FDA) for the treatment of anxiety disorders. The SSRIs approved by the FDA for the treatment of various anxiety disorders, include the following:

- Fluoxetine (Prozac, generics)
- Fluvoxamine (Luvox, generics)
- Paroxetine (Paxil, generics; Paxil CR)
- Sertraline (Zoloft, generics)
- Escitalopram (Lexapro)

The SNRIs approved by the FDA for the treatment of anxiety disorders include the following:

- Venlafaxine extended release (Effexor XR)
- Duloxetine (Cymbalta)

The benzodiazepines approved by the FDA for the treatment of anxiety and various anxiety disorders include the following:

- Alprazolam (Xanax, generics; Xanax XR)
- Clonazepam (Klonopin, generics)
- Lorazepam (Ativan, generics)
- Diazepam (Valium, generics)
- Chlordiazepoxide (Librium, generics)
- Oxazepam (Serax)
- Clorazepate (Tranxene, generics)

The nonbenzodiazepine 5-HT1A receptor agonist medications approved by the FDA for the treatment of anxiety disorders include the following:

- Buspirone (BuSpar, generics)

Other medications useful for the treatment of anxiety disorders include beta-blockers, tricyclic and other antidepressants, anticonvulsant medications, atypical antipsychotics, antihistamines, and monoamine oxidase (MAO) inhibitors. Many of these medications are used off-label for the treatment of anxiety disorders, especially with difficult cases, and have anecdotal clinical as well as scientific literature to support their use.

Education
Psychoeducation is a vital part of the treatment of anxiety disorders. It is important to help the patient understand the disorder, both psychologically and medically. For example, helping the patient to understand that substances such as caffeine, illicit drugs, and some over-the-counter (OTC) cold medications can cause or exacerbate anxiety symptoms can go a long way in the effective management of anxiety disorders. Sharing information such as discussing direct-to-consumer advertising messages or information from appropriate Internet sites can be extremely helpful. Support and reassurance is invaluable. Handouts such as pamphlets describing the disorder in more detail allow patients to read the information at a time when they are more relaxed and their concentration is perhaps better. Close follow-up by phone and office visits is imperative, especially early in the treatment.

Principles of Psychopharmacotherapy
It is extremely important to give the initial treatment a fair trial. Ensuring that therapeutic dosages are utilized and that an appropriate length of treatment (e.g., medications, psychotherapy) is undertaken, and monitoring for side effects are mandatory. Trying

TABLE 1.5. Psychopharmacotherapy: principles for primary care

- The diagnostic assessment is fundamental and may be revised
- Complete recovery generally requires more than pharmacotherapy alone
- The phase of an illness is important regarding initial treatment and the duration of treatment (e.g., acute, continuation, and maintenance)
- One must always consider the risk-to-benefit ratio regarding the treatment strategy
- When selecting a medication regimen, consider comorbid disorders
- First-line choice of medication for initial treatment includes consideration of family history regarding a response (good or bad) to a specific agent, especially for a similar disorder
- First-line choice of medication for a subsequent episode includes consideration of prior personal and family history regarding a response (good or bad) to a specific agent
- Determine and monitor specific symptoms that serve as markers for the disorder (outcome measures) over the course of treatment
- Monitor for the development of adverse effects throughout the course of treatment and utilize appropriate laboratory to ensure optimal efficacy as well as safety
- Remember that when stopped, many antidepressant medications may cause discontinuation symptoms, especially if stopped too quickly

Adapted from ref. [23].

other therapeutic approaches if the current method of treatment is unsuccessful can be helpful.

Janicak et al. [23] suggested several general principles for decision making with regard to psychopharmacotherapy in clinical practice (Table 1.5). These principles are applicable for the treatment of anxiety disorders by the primary care practitioner.

When to Seek Assistance from a Mental Health Professional
Primary care practitioners evaluate and treat a large percentage of patients with anxiety disorders. Other health professionals, including dentists, also treat many patients who suffer from anxiety disorders, and it is imperative that they recognize these disorders and ensure that the patient's anxiety symptoms are managed appropriately. It is important for all primary care practitioners to become familiar with the common anxiety disorders and their treatment. As with any profession, however, it is important to know one's limits and not exceed them.

Often, consultation with or referral to a mental health professional is necessary for the comprehensive management of complex patients with anxiety disorders. Seeking assistance is acceptable and prudent, and is to be encouraged. Psychiatrists, psychologists, social workers, and counselors can be a valuable part of the health care team. The ideal scenario for the comprehensive management of anxiety disorders is a primary care practitioner who has a good working relationship with mental health professionals and is in close proximity for consultation and referral. In the following situations, consultation/referral may be indicated:

- Anxiety disorders requiring higher dosages or complex combinations of medications
- Comorbid conditions including other anxiety or psychiatric disorders such as bipolar disorder and psychotic disorders
- Suicidal behaviors
- Cases requiring specialized training in CBT or other psychotherapies
- Cases requiring group therapy or self-help therapy groups
- Patients requesting follow-up with clergy

The availability of services can be an issue in some areas, and so at times the primary care practitioner may have to do it all—at least for a while! Recognizing, diagnosing, and managing patients with anxiety disorders can be a difficult but most rewarding experience. The information in this pocket guide will make this experience more comfortable.

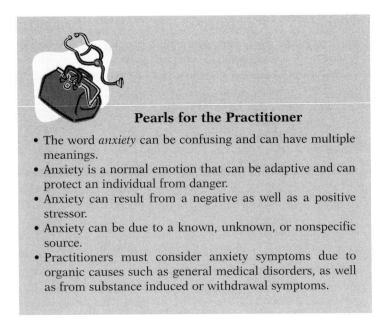

Pearls for the Practitioner

- The word *anxiety* can be confusing and can have multiple meanings.
- Anxiety is a normal emotion that can be adaptive and can protect an individual from danger.
- Anxiety can result from a negative as well as a positive stressor.
- Anxiety can be due to a known, unknown, or nonspecific source.
- Practitioners must consider anxiety symptoms due to organic causes such as general medical disorders, as well as from substance induced or withdrawal symptoms.

- Anxiety becomes pathological in the form of anxiety disorders when there is marked distress, impairment in functioning, and avoidance behaviors.
- Anxiety disorders are often comorbid with other anxiety disorders, other psychiatric disorders, and general medical disorders.
- Common neurotransmitters associated with the anxiety disorders include serotonin, norepinephrine, and GABA.
- Screening instruments can be helpful in providing clinically relevant information to assist with anxiety disorder diagnosis and management.
- Treatment of the anxiety disorders includes pharmacotherapy, psychotherapy, and psychoeducation.

References

1. Venes D, ed. Taber's Cyclopedic Medical Dictionary, 20th ed., Philadelphia: F.A. Davis, 2005.
2. Shader RI, Greenblatt DJ. Approaches to the treatment of anxiety states. In: Shader RI, ed. Manual of Psychiatric Therapeutics, 3rd ed. Philadelphia: Lippincott Williams & Wilkins, 2003:184–209.
3. Foa EB, Andrews LW. Anxiety disorders: where they are, where do they come from. In: Jamieson P, ed. If Your Adolescent Has an Anxiety Disorder. New York: Oxford University Press, 2006:9–41.
4. Ninan PT. The functional anatomy, neurochemistry, and pharmacology of anxiety. J Clin Psychiatry 1999;60(suppl 22):12–17.
5. McGregor JC, Anxiety disorders. In: Rakel RE, Bope ET, eds. Conn's Current Therapy, Philadelphia: Saunders, 2006:1345–1350.
6. Kessler RC, Berglund P, Demler O, Jin R, Walters EE. Lifetime prevalence and age-of onset distributions of DSM-IV disorders in the national comorbidity survey replication. Arch Gen Psychiatry 2005;62:593–602.
7. National Institute of Mental Health. Anxiety disorders. http://www.nimh.nih.gov/publicat/anxiety.cfm.
8. Wang PS, Lane M, Olfson M, Pincus HA, Wells KB, Kessler RC. Twelve-month use of mental health services in the United States. Arch Gen Psychiatry 2005;62:629–640.
9. American Psychiatric Association. Diagnostic and Statistical Manual of Mental Disorders, 4th ed., text revision. Washington, DC: American Psychiatric Association, 2000.
10. Charney DS. Anxiety disorders: introduction and overview. In: Sadock BJ, Sadock VA, eds. Sadock's Comprehensive Textbook of Psychiatry, 8th ed., vol. 1. Philadelphia: Lippincott Williams & Wilkins, 2005:1718–1719.
11. Cahill SP, Foa EB. Anxiety disorders: cognitive-behavioral therapy. In: Sadock BJ, Sadock VA, eds. Sadock's Comprehensive Textbook of Psychiatry, 8th ed., vol. 1. Philadelphia: Lippincott Williams & Wilkins, 2005:1788–1799.

12. McMahon FJ, Kassem L. Anxiety disorders: genetics. In: Sadock BJ, Sadock VA, eds. Sadock's Comprehensive Textbook of Psychiatry, 8th ed., vol. 1. Philadelphia: Lippincott Williams & Wilkins, 2005:1759–1761.
13. Nemiah JC. Anxiety disorders: psychodynamic aspects. In: Sadock BJ, Sadock VA, eds. Sadock's Comprehensive Textbook of Psychiatry, 8th ed., vol. 1. Philadelphia: Lippincott Williams & Wilkins, 2005: 1762–1767.
14. Neumeister A, Bonne O, Charney DS. Anxiety disorders: neurochemical aspects. In: Sadock BJ, Sadock VA, eds. Sadock's Comprehensive Textbook of Psychiatry, 8th ed., vol. 1. Philadelphia: Lippincott Williams & Wilkins, 2005:1739–1747.
15. Hollifield M, Mackey A, Davidson J. Integrating therapies for anxiety disorders. Psychiatr Ann 2006;36[5]:331–338.
16. Drevets WC, Charney DS. Anxiety disorders: Neuroimaging. In: Sadock BJ, Sadock VA, eds. Sadock's Comprehensive Textbook of Psychiatry, 8th ed., vol. 1. Philadelphia: Lippincott Williams & Wilkins, 2005:1748–1757.
17. Grillon C. Anxiety disorders: psychophysiological aspects. In: Sadock BJ, Sadock VA, eds. Sadock's Comprehensive Textbook of Psychiatry, 8th ed., vol. 1. Philadelphia: Lippincott Williams & Wilkins, 2005:1728–1738.
18. Stein MB. Anxiety disorders: somatic treatment. In: Sadock BJ, Sadock VA, eds. Sadock's Comprehensive Textbook of Psychiatry, 8th ed., vol. 1. Philadelphia: Lippincott Williams & Wilkins, 2005:1780–1787.
19. Pine DS, McClure EB. Anxiety disorders: clinical features. In: Sadock BJ, Sadock VA, eds. Sadock's Comprehensive Textbook of Psychiatry, 8th ed., vol. 1. Philadelphia: Lippincott Williams & Wilkins, 2005:1768–1779.
20. Frei R. Anxiety disorders are warning signs for physical disorders, and vice versa. CNS News 2006;9[5]:1,36.
21. Merikangas KR. Anxiety disorders: epidemiology. In: Sadock BJ, Sadock VA, eds. Sadock's Comprehensive Textbook of Psychiatry, 8th ed., vol. 1. Philadelphia: Lippincott Williams & Wilkins, 2005:1720–1727.
22. Davidson J. Managing anxiety disorders: psychopharmacologic treatment options. Psychiatric Times April 2006;23:80,82–83.
23. Janicak PG, Davis JM, Preskorn SH, Ayd FJ. Principles of pharmacotherapy. In: Retford DC, ed. Principles and Practice of Psychopharmacotherapy. Baltimore: Williams & Wilkins, 1993:1–28.

2
Brief Psychiatric History and Mental Status Examination

John R. Vanin

A comprehensive medical evaluation includes a thorough history, physical examination, and appropriate laboratory, imaging and other studies. An important portion of the history in a primary care evaluation is the psychiatric history and the mental status examination. When evaluating a patient for mental or emotional disorders, history is truly everything. Often, the practitioner must ask specific questions to assess the presence of common mental disorders in order to supplement other information or because the patient does not recognize or does not volunteer the symptoms.

Casting ones net for the symptoms of common mental disorders, including the category of anxiety disorders, is extremely helpful to fully assess a patient's emotional and physical status. Disorders that comorbidly occur may further complicate matters, especially if common symptoms are shared. For example, shared symptoms of both generalized anxiety disorder and major depressive disorder include worrying, poor concentration, insomnia, fatigue, irritability, and somatic concerns. An appropriate diagnosis and treatment plan can be instituted only after the clinical symptoms and signs are fully recognized and evaluated.

The information in this book is applicable to evaluations of adult patients, age 18 years or older, although sections may be applicable to younger patients. The information is based on scholarly information supported by research and practical suggestions based on cumulative clinical experiences of the authors.

EVALUATING ANXIETY DISORDERS

Anxiety disorders are the most prevalent mental disorders in the general population [1]. They are a family of related but distinct disorders. Anxiety disorders are complex disorders and may be difficult to recognize and treat, especially if there are comorbid problems such as depression and substance abuse. There are no distinctively characteristic markers to make a presumptive diagnosis of an anxiety disorder despite an abundance of physiologic symptoms [1]. Psychophysiology, a noninvasive tool dealing with the correlation of the mind and body, historically has relied on electrical signals generated by the body and recorded by way of electrodes on the scalp, hands, and face. It is used to quantify normal and abnormal physiological activity and reactivity [2]. In addition to measures such as palmar sweating, respiration, heart rate, blood pressure, and reflexes, psychophysiology has incorporated neuroendocrine physiology and brain imaging such as positron emission tomography (PET) [2]. It is interesting to note that despite physiological symptoms playing a crucial role in the diagnostic profile of anxiety disorders, the evaluation of symptoms and the formal diagnosis are based primarily on verbal self-reports. Physiological measures have the potential to help objectively assess and better characterize anxiety symptoms and identify psychological and neurobiological dysfunctions [2]. Psychophysiology essentially remains a research tool, however, regarding the causes and nature of anxiety.

DIAGNOSIS OF ANXIETY DISORDERS

The diagnosis of anxiety disorders continues to depend on the clinical interview, which utilizes self-reports of symptoms as well as observation of objective signs of anxiety. An index of suspicion is often helpful in assessing the presence of an anxiety disorder. For example, a patient may not present with the classic symptoms such as excessive hand-washing rituals in obsessive-compulsive disorder. Instead, severe obsessive thinking and perhaps checking rituals may be present, and the patient fails to mention these symptoms to the examiner. Clinical experience has shown that several psychiatric disorders, including social anxiety disorder, obsessive-compulsive disorder, posttraumatic stress disorder, as well as bipolar disorder and adult attention-deficit/hyperactivity disorder, commonly occur, may not readily present themselves, and are easily missed. It is interesting to note that three of these five easily unrecognized disorders are categories of anxiety disorders!

The subtypes of the anxiety disorders are defined by the standardized diagnostic criteria of the American Psychiatric Association's *Diagnostic and Statistical Manual of Mental Disorders,* 4th edition, text revision (DSM-IV-TR) [3]. Table 2.1 lists the categories of DSM-IV-TR anxiety disorders [3]. Tables 2.2 through 2.9 list the key features of the common anxiety disorders [1,3]. Although adjustment disorder with anxiety is not a formal anxiety disorder in the DSM-IV-TR, it is an important disorder to recognize

TABLE 2.1. DSM-IV-TR anxiety disorder categories

- Adjustment disorder with anxiety*
- Panic disorder (with/without agoraphobia)
- Phobic disorders
  - Agoraphobia**
  - Specific phobia
  - Social phobia (social anxiety disorder)
- Obsessive-compulsive disorder
- Acute stress disorder
- Posttraumatic stress disorder
- Generalized anxiety disorder
- Anxiety disorder due to a general medical condition
- Substance-induced anxiety disorder
- Anxiety disorder not otherwise specified

*Not a formal DSM-IV-TR anxiety disorder.
**Not a DSM-IV-TR codable disorder.
Adapted from ref. [3].

TABLE 2.2. Key features of panic disorder

- Recurrent unexpected panic attacks
- Persistent concern about additional attacks
- Worry about the meaning of or the consequences of the attacks (e.g., heart attack, stroke, "going crazy")
- Significant change in behavior related to the attacks (e.g., avoiding places)
- With or without presence of agoraphobia

Adapted from refs. [1] and [3].

TABLE 2.3. Key features of agoraphobia

- Anxiety about being in places or situations from which escape might be difficult, embarrassing, or in which help may not be available in the event of having a panic attack
- Places and situations are avoided or endured with anxiety or distress

Adapted from refs. [1] and [3].

TABLE 2.4. Key features of specific phobia

- Marked and persistent fear that is excessive, unreasonable, and brought on by the presence or anticipation of a specific object or situation
- Exposure provokes an immediate anxiety response
- Recognition that the fear is excessive or unreasonable
- Phobic stimulus is avoided or endured with distress
- Avoidance, anticipatory anxiety, or distress is significantly impairing

Adapted from refs. [1] and [3].

TABLE 2.5. Key features of social phobia (social anxiety disorder)

- Marked and persistent fear of one or more social or performance situations in which the person is concerned about negative evaluation or scrutiny by others
- Recognition that the fear is excessive or unreasonable
- Fears acting in a way or showing anxiety symptoms that will be humiliating or embarrassing
- Feared social or performance situations are avoided or endured with intense anxiety or distress

Adapted from refs. [1] and [3].

TABLE 2.6. Key features of obsessive-compulsive disorder

- Experiencing obsessions or compulsions
- Recognition that the obsessions or compulsions are excessive or unreasonable
- Obsessions or compulsions cause much distress, are time-consuming, or cause significant interference in daily functioning

Adapted from refs. [1] and [3].

TABLE 2.7. Key features of acute stress disorder

- Exposure to a traumatic event
- Individual experiences dissociative symptoms
- Traumatic event is persistently reexperienced
- Marked symptoms of anxiety and increased arousal
- Marked avoidance of stimuli that arouse trauma recollection
- Disturbance occurs within 4 weeks of the traumatic event, lasts for a minimum of 2 days and a maximum of 4 weeks
- Disturbance causes significant distress or impairment in daily functioning

Adapted from ref. [3].

TABLE 2.8. Key features of posttraumatic stress disorder

- Exposure to a traumatic event
- Traumatic event is persistently reexperienced
- Persistent avoidance of stimuli associated with the trauma and numbing of general responsiveness
- Persistent symptoms of increased arousal
- Duration of the disturbance is more than 1 month
- Disturbance causes significant distress or impairment in daily functioning

Adapted from refs. [1] and [3].

TABLE 2.9. Key features of generalized anxiety disorder

- Excessive anxiety and worry about a number of events or activities for at least 6 months
- Difficulty controlling the worry
- Anxiety and worry associated with additional symptoms, including somatic
- Anxiety, worry, physical symptoms cause significant distress or impairment in daily functioning

Adapted from ref. [3].

and evaluate in primary care. For conditions that approach but do not fulfill diagnostic criteria for a major psychiatric disorder, diagnostic and treatment decisions rely on a practitioner's clinical judgment [4]. This certainly applies to the anxiety disorders as well. Subthreshold conditions are important to recognize and evaluate, especially if they impact personal, social, occupational, and academic functioning. The current diagnostic criteria for many mental disorders include the stipulation that the disturbance causes clinically significant distress or impairment in social, occupational, or other important areas of functioning. Some clinicians feel that suffering from the diagnostic symptoms may be sufficient for a diagnosis at times, even before functional disturbances appear. Treatment may not be necessary at the time but monitoring may be warranted.

The careful evaluation of the patient by the primary care practitioner regarding anxiety symptoms is important for comprehensive care. The recognition and management of anxiety disorders, either individually or comorbidly, is important for the patient's quality of life. Distinguishing the common anxiety disorders from each other and other psychiatric and general medical disorders can be significant regarding treatment decisions. The practitioner and the patient may never know if an anxiety disorder is present unless specific screening questions are asked about each specific anxiety disorder category. A patient may not volunteer the symptoms of an anxiety disorder initially as the chief complaint or even after a few open-ended questions are asked. Closed-ended questions are often necessary to actively screen for the common anxiety disorders.

SCREENING FOR ANXIETY DISORDERS

Formal screening guidelines and suggestions for anxiety disorders are practically nonexistent [5]. Representative common anxiety disorder screening questions for the busy practitioner are listed in Tables 2.10 to 2.15 [6,7]. Many questions are adapted from

TABLE 2.10. Screening questions for generalized anxiety disorder

- Have there been days at a time when you felt extremely tense, anxious, or nervous for no special reason?
  If yes: Have you felt this way even when you were at home with nothing to do?
  If yes: Have these anxious or nervous feelings bothered you for at least 6 months?
  If yes: Practitioner should further evaluate for generalized anxiety disorder

Adapted from ref. [6].

TABLE 2.11. Screening questions for adjustment disorder with anxiety

- Have you been worried or upset about something that happened to you in the past 3 months? For example, loss of a job, separation, divorce, accident, death of a loved one.
  If yes: Compared to most people, do you feel you had more trouble handling this situation? (e.g., nervousness, worry)
  If yes: Practitioner should further evaluate for adjustment disorder with anxiety

Adapted from ref. [6].

TABLE 2.12. Screening questions for panic disorder

- Have you ever had sudden spells or attacks of fear, nervousness, or panic, that seem to come on all of a sudden, out of the blue for no particular reason?
  If yes: Did you have these attacks even though a health care practitioner said there was nothing seriously wrong with you?
  Another screening question which we find very useful is:
- Does your heart ever beat really fast, and you feel short of breath, light headed, and feel like you have to get out of a place or situation immediately?
- If yes: Practitioner should further evaluate for panic disorder

Adapted from ref. [6].

well-researched screening questions that can help a practitioner recognize and further evaluate anxiety disorders in daily practice. If a patient answers in the affirmative for any of the screening questions, further in-depth evaluation of that particular disorder should be pursued. The Anxiety and Depression Detector, a recently developed, brief five-item screening device for anxiety and depressive disorders in primary care settings is listed in Figure 2.1 [5]. This screening instrument may be particularly helpful for comorbid

TABLE 2.13. Screening questions for phobic disorders

- Have you ever been much more afraid of things or situations than the average person? (e.g., flying, heights, needles, animals, thunder, sight of blood).
- Despite knowing it was safe, have you ever been so afraid to leave home by yourself that you would not go?
- Have you ever been afraid to go into places like supermarkets or elevators because you were afraid of not being able to get out?
- Have you ever been so afraid of embarrassing yourself that you would not do certain things in public? (e.g., speaking out in a room full of people, eating in a restaurant, using a public restroom)
- If yes to any of the above: Did you ever try to avoid the feared object or situation whenever you could?
  If yes: Practitioner should further evaluate for phobic disorder

Adapted from ref. [6].

TABLE 2.14. Screening questions for obsessive-compulsive disorder

- Have you ever been bothered by certain thoughts, images, or impulses that came into your mind repeatedly even though you tried to ignore or stop them?
  If yes: Describe the thoughts, images or impulses
- Have you ever felt you had to repeat a certain act over and over even when this action did not seem to make much sense? (e.g., checking or counting things over and over again; arranging objects in a certain way; washing your hands over and over again although you knew they were clean)
  If yes: Practitioner should further evaluate for obsessive-compulsive disorder

Adapted from ref. [6].

TABLE 2.15. Screening questions for posttraumatic stress disorder (PTSD) (primary care PTSD screen)

In your life, have you ever had any experience that was so frightening, horrible, or upsetting that, in the past month, you...
- Have had nightmares about it or thought about it when you did not want to?
- Tried hard not to think about the experience or went out of your way to avoid situations that reminded you of it?
- Were constantly on guard, watchful, or easily startled?
- Felt numb or detached from others, activities, or your surroundings?
  If yes to any three items, screen is positive: Practitioner should further evaluate for posttraumatic stress disorder

Adapted from ref. [7]. Public Domain.

Name_____ Date_____
In the past 3 months...

1. Did you ever have a spell or an attack when all of a sudden you felt frightened, anxious, or very uneasy? Yes No
2. Would you say that you have been bothered by "nerves" or feeling anxious or on edge? Yes No
3. Would you say that being anxious or uncomfortable around other people is a problem in your life? Yes No
4. Did you have a period of one week or more when you lost interest in most things like work, hobbies, and other things you usually enjoyed? Yes No
5. Some people have terrible experiences happen to them, like being attacked or threatened with a weapon; being in a fire or a bad traffic accident; being sexually assaulted; or seeing someone being badly injured or killed. Has anything like this ever happened to you? Yes No

If Yes:
In the past three months, have you had recurrent dreams or nightmares about this experience, or recurrent thoughts or "flashbacks" (times when you felt as though it was happening again, even though it wasn't)? Yes No
Note: A yes answer to any of the items 1 through 4 or the second part of item 5 is considered a positive screen. Further evaluate for panic disorder, generalized anxiety disorder, social anxiety disorder, major depressive disorder, posttraumatic stress disorder. (Note: This figure is in the public domain.)

FIGURE 2.1. The Anxiety and Depression Detector.

anxiety and depressive disorders, which are very prevalent conditions. Clinicians must use their clinical judgment regarding the use of additional screening questions, especially if the patient answers in the negative and there is a suspicion of an undisclosed anxiety disorder.

ANXIETY DISORDERS AND GENERAL MEDICAL DISORDERS
One must keep in mind that general medical disorders can cause symptoms of an anxiety disorder, and primary anxiety disorders can mimic a general medical disorder. The effects of medications prescribed for a general medical condition as well as over-the-counter, herbal, and other nonprescribed substances can mimic an anxiety disorder. The treatment of a general medical disorder can complicate the course and treatment of anxiety disorders and vice

versa. In addition, the primary care practitioner must monitor for drug interactions, including those involving the cytochrome P-450 enzyme system.

BRIEF PSYCHIATRIC EVALUATION

The psychiatric evaluation performed in a busy primary care practice need not be long or complex. A comprehensive but concise history and mental status examination will often provide the necessary information for a good differential diagnosis and treatment plan. The differential diagnosis is subject to revisions as information becomes available or as a disorder evolves. The following Primary Care Psychiatric Evaluation Guideline (PCPEG) contains the components of a thorough psychiatric evaluation for primary care practitioners (Fig. 2.2). This evaluation guideline is a format

Name_____Date_____Age_____Sex_____Marital status_____
Chief complaint_____

History of present illness_____

Depressive disorder (unipolar, dysthymia)_____

Bipolar disorder (depression, mania, mixed, rapid cycling)_____

Anxiety disorders (generalized, panic, obsessive-compulsive, social/
performance, posttraumatic stress)_____

Psychotic disorder (hallucinations, delusions, ideas of reference)___

Adult attention-deficit hyperactivity disorder_____

Substance-induced symptoms_____

Symptoms secondary to a general medical condition_____

Personality characteristics_____

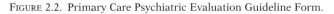

FIGURE 2.2. Primary Care Psychiatric Evaluation Guideline Form.

Past history
Psychiatric_____

General medical_____

Neurological (closed head injury, loss of consciousness, seizures)___

Medications (prescribed, over-the-counter)_____

Alternative treatments (supplements, herbal)_____

Allergies (medication, other)_____

Substance use (alcohol, nicotine, caffeine, inappropriate prescription use, illicit drugs)_____

Personal/social history
Developmental_____
Education_____
Occupational_____
Relationships_____
Sexual_____
Trauma/abuse_____
Involvement with social agencies/court system_____
Suicide/homicide_____
Family history
Mother_____
Father_____
Siblings_____
Grandparents_____
Children_____
Review of systems
General_____

Sleep_____
Appetite/diet_____
Exercise_____

FIGURE 2.2. Continued.

Mental status examination_____
_____
_____
_____
_____
_____
_____
Physical examination_____
_____
Laboratory/studies_____
_____
Assessment/differential diagnosis
Axis I_____
Axis II_____
Axis III_____
Axis IV_____
Axis V_____
Treatment plan_____

FIGURE 2.2. *Continued*.

that we developed and is commonly used for mental health clinical evaluations at the West Virginia University Student Health Service by primary care practitioners, psychiatrists, residents, and students, and may be reproduced by the practitioner. Citation of the source is appreciated. The level of detail varies as one utilizes this guideline, depending on the patient's problem and the skills and clinical judgment of the practitioner. Much of the evaluation is standard with regard to a comprehensive general medical evaluation, with an emphasis on the standard principles of psychiatric diagnosis, mental status examination, and treatment planning. The mental health aspects are based on the American Psychiatric Association's Practice Guideline for Psychiatric Evaluation of Adults [4].

PSYCHIATRIC HISTORY
The psychiatric history includes the following information about the patient: the chief complaint; present illness; pertinent past history; personal, social, and family history; and the mental status examination (MSE). The MSE is a systematic collection of information based on the patient's behavior, sensorium, and cognitive function [4, 8, 9]. The practitioner utilizes the MSE to obtain evidence of current symptoms of a mental disorder. The categories of the MSE obtained via observation, listening, and formal mental status testing are listed in Table 2.16 [4, 8, 9].

TABLE 2.16. Mental status examination

- Appearance and behavior
- Motor activity (e.g., tremors, nail-biting, restlessness)
- Attitude (e.g., cooperativeness, guarded, embarrassment)
- Speech (e.g., volume, tone, rate, coherence)
- Mood
- Affect
- Thought content and perceptions
  - Worries
  - Obsessions
  - Impulses
  - Phobias
  - Delusions
  - Hallucinations
  - Suicide/homicide
  - Other forms of disordered thinking
- Cognitive status
  - Attention and concentration
  - Level of consciousness
  - Orientation
  - Memory (immediate, recent, remote)
  - Fund of knowledge
  - Abstraction
  - Judgment
  - Insight
  - Language
  - Executive function
  - Calculation
  - Drawing

Adapted from refs. [4], [8], and [9].

To be most effective, a practitioner must develop a comfortable style to gather the pertinent information, exhibiting sensitivity, compassion, and empathy. Making eye contact is important, especially while taking notes. This also applies to electronic medical recording of information. Listening carefully and noting the patient's nonverbal responses and behaviors (e.g., blushing, sighing, hair twisting, leg-shaking, finger-picking, tearfulness) are extremely helpful techniques in history taking.

ANXIETY DISORDER SCREENING INSTRUMENTS

Anxiety disorder screening tools are available to assist the practitioner in assessing anxiety disorders in the clinical setting. Examples of several of the measures are listed in Tables 2.17 to 2.23 [10–14]. Some of the screening tools are more practical than others for the

TABLE 2.17. Features of the Hamilton Rating Scale for Anxiety (HAM-A)

- Assesses somatic and cognitive anxiety symptoms
- Extensively used to monitor treatment responses of generalized anxiety disorder in studies and in clinical settings
- Limited coverage of worry; does not include episodic anxiety
- 14 items, rated 0–4 on an unanchored severity scale
- Designed to be administered by a clinician
- Total score range 0–56
- Formal training or use of structured guide required for high reliability
- Validity limited by lack of coverage of areas critical to the modern understanding of anxiety disorders

Adapted from ref. [10].

TABLE 2.18. Features of the Posttraumatic Stress Disorder Scale: clinician administered PTSD scale (CAPS)

- Clinician administered
- 17 items, 5-point scale (0–4)
- Administered by a trained clinician; requires 45–60 minutes to complete
- Demonstrated reliability and validity
- In the public domain, but generally too lengthy for use in clinician practice

Adapted from ref. [10].

TABLE 2.19. Features of Yale-Brown Obsessive-Compulsive Scale (YBOCS)

- Measures severity of symptoms in obsessive-compulsive disorder and may be used to clinically monitor treatment response (copyrighted)
- 64-item checklist administered before YBOCS to provide detailed assessment of specific content of patient's symptoms
- 10 items rated on a semistructured interview: 5 on obsessions/5 on compulsions
- Self-administered version available
- Item-specific anchors, scored from 0–4
- Overall total score range from 0–40
- Can be completed in ≤15 minutes
- Good reliability and good validity

Adapted from ref. [10].

busy clinician. In addition to initially helping with diagnosis, screening instruments can be utilized to follow a patient's progress. Further information on screening measures is provided in the individual anxiety disorder chapters.

TABLE 2.20. Features of Panic Disorder Severity Scale (PDSS)

- Brief rating scale of panic disorder severity
- 7 items, rated on item-specific Likert scale 0–4
- Total score range 0–28
- Designed for clinicians; patient scored computerized version available
- Reliability excellent; validity supported by correlation with other anxiety measures
- Useful for monitoring panic disorder in clinical practice

Adapted from ref. [10].

TABLE 2.21. Features of Beck Anxiety Inventory (BAI)

- Screening device for discriminating anxiety from depression and assessing the severity of the anxiety symptoms
- Useful in assessing anxiety in clinical and research settings
- 21 items on common anxiety symptoms; patient rates symptom intensity on 0–3 scale
- Administration and scoring are rapid; total score range 0–63
- Adequately covers major cognitive, affective, and physiological anxiety symptoms
- Reliability—excellent; validity—appropriate convergent and discriminate

Adapted from refs. [11] and [12].

TABLE 2.22. Features of Social Phobia Inventory (SPIN)

- 17-item self-rating scale
- Each item rated 0–4; total score ranging from 0–68
- Measures fear, phobic avoidance, and autonomic symptoms
- Can be used to distinguish between those with and without social anxiety disorder

Adapted from ref. [13].

TABLE 2.23. Features of Liebowitz Social Anxiety Scale (LSAS)

- Screening test for social anxiety disorder (copyrighted)
- Assesses range of social interaction and performance situations that patients with social phobia fear and/or avoid
- 24-item clinician-rating scale divided into two subscales: social interactional and performance situations
- Patient rates fear and avoidance on 0–3 Likert scale

Adapted from ref. [14].

The PCPEG can be helpful for the busy primary care clinician. The handy format (Figure 2.2) based on the following descriptions is available in the Pocket Guide for copying and practical use.

PRIMARY CARE PSYCHIATRIC EVALUATION GUIDELINE (PCPEG)

Chief Complaint/Reason for Evaluation
Early open-ended questions may be helpful: "What has been troubling you?" "What led you to come in for help?" "What brings you in today?"

History of Present Illness
- Depressive disorders
- Bipolar disorder
- Anxiety disorders
- Psychotic disorders
- Adult attention deficit hyperactivity disorder
- Substance-induced symptoms
- Symptoms secondary to a general medical disorder

It is very helpful to screen each patient specifically for the above categories. It is also appropriate to assess a patient's personality or characterological features.

Appropriate treatment, including psychological as well as pharmacotherapy, works best if a hierarchy of the most severe disorders to the least severe is determined and treated accordingly. Clinicians must use their judgment regarding the order in the hierarchy. For example, let's take a patient with the diagnosis of substance abuse, bipolar disorder, social anxiety disorder and adult attention-deficit hyperactivity disorder (ADHD). An effective management approach would be initially to control the substance abuse and bipolar symptoms, and then manage the social anxiety symptoms and adult attention deficit manifestations. After removing substances of abuse and stabilizing mood swings, more effective management of anxiety disorder and ADHD symptoms can occur.

Past History
Psychiatric
General medical/surgical
Neurological (closed head injury, loss of consciousness, seizure disorder)

Current Medications
Prescribed
Oral contraceptives
Over-the-counter
Vitamins
Supplements
Weight control
Herbal products

Allergies
To medications
Others

Substance Use
Alcohol
Nicotine
Caffeine
Inappropriate prescription use
Illicit drugs

Personal/Social History
Developmental
Education
Occupational
Trauma/Abuse
Sexual
Involvement with social agencies/court system
Relationships
Suicidal/homicidal behavior

Family History

Review of Systems
General
Sleep
Appetite

Physical Examination
The general medical condition of a patient is important to assess as part of a psychiatric evaluation. A physical examination allows the practitioner to properly assess the potential cause of the patient's psychiatric symptoms (e.g., anxiety symptoms) and the need for general medical care, and to make choices regarding the treatment, especially regarding medications [4]. Laboratory and other diagnostic

tests may be helpful in a psychiatric evaluation to establish or exclude a diagnosis, assist in the choice of treatment, or to monitor treatment and side effects [4]. For example, thyroid function tests are indicated if the practitioner suspects a thyroid disorder is related to the patients anxiety symptoms. Urine drug screens are useful for substance use disorders. Brain imaging may help determine the presence of a structural neurological abnormality causing psychiatric symptoms such as a stroke or tumor.

There are no general guidelines regarding "routine" tests for a psychiatric evaluation. Each patient should be considered individually, and the tests ordered are based on the setting, the clinical presentation, the potential treatment, and patient preferences [4]. Table 2.24 lists examples of diagnostic tests that may helpful as part of a primary care general psychiatric evaluation.

Mental Status Examination

Information gathered in the general history and via observation often includes much of the mental status examination. One may need to supplement specific areas, however. The degree of formal mental status testing depends on patient requirements (Table 2.16) [4, 8, 9].

Functional Assessment/Differential Diagnosis

Treatment Plan

Diagnostic tests (e.g., laboratory, imaging, electrophysiologic) Psychoeducation (includes written material such as pamphlets, other patient information)

TABLE 2.24. General psychiatric evaluation: common diagnostic tests

- Laboratory (e.g., CBC, comprehensive metabolic panel, lipid panel, RPR, urinalysis, drug abuse screen, TSH, serum medication concentration)
- ECG, Holter monitoring
- EEG
- CT scan
- MRI
- Tests of other medical conditions (e.g. HIV)
- Psychological testing

CBC, complete blood count; CT, computed tomography; ECG, electrocardiogram; EEG, electroencephalogram; HIV, human immunodeficiency virus; MRI, magnetic resonance imaging; RPR, rapid plasma reagin; TSH, thyroid-stimulating hormone.

Medications (includes discussion of consent and side effects)
Psychotherapy
Consultation/referral (e.g., psychiatrist/psychologist, psychotherapist, clergy, disability services agency)
Follow-up planning

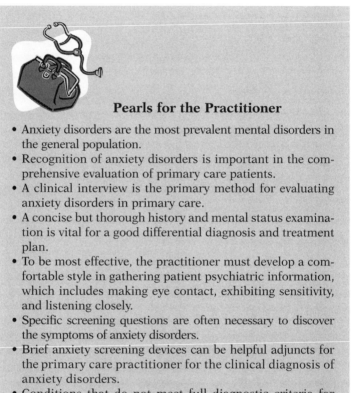

Pearls for the Practitioner

- Anxiety disorders are the most prevalent mental disorders in the general population.
- Recognition of anxiety disorders is important in the comprehensive evaluation of primary care patients.
- A clinical interview is the primary method for evaluating anxiety disorders in primary care.
- A concise but thorough history and mental status examination is vital for a good differential diagnosis and treatment plan.
- To be most effective, the practitioner must develop a comfortable style in gathering patient psychiatric information, which includes making eye contact, exhibiting sensitivity, and listening closely.
- Specific screening questions are often necessary to discover the symptoms of anxiety disorders.
- Brief anxiety screening devices can be helpful adjuncts for the primary care practitioner for the clinical diagnosis of anxiety disorders.
- Conditions that do not meet full diagnostic criteria for anxiety disorders are important to recognize and evaluate.

References

1. Merikangas KR. Anxiety disorders: epidemiology. In: Sadock BJ, Sadock VA, eds. Sadocks's Comprehensive Textbook of Psychiatry, 8th ed., vol. 1. Philadelphia: Lippincott Williams & Wilkins, 2005:1720–1728.
2. Grillon C. Anxiety disorders: psychophysiological aspects. In: Sadock BJ, Sadock VA, eds. Sadock's Comprehensive Textbook of Psychiatry, 8th ed., vol. 1. Philadelphia: Lippincott Williams & Wilkins, 1728–1739.

3. American Psychiatric Association. Diagnostic and Statistical Manual of Mental Disorders, 4th ed., text revision. Washington, DC: American Psychiatric Association, 2000.
4. American Psychiatric Association. Practice Guidelines for Psychiatric Evaluation of Adults, 1995. http://www.psych.org/psych_pract/treatg/pg/pg_adult.cfm?pf=y.
5. Means-Christensen AJ, Sherbourne CD, Roy-Byrne PP, Craske MG, Stein MB. Using five questions to screen for five common mental disorders in primary care: diagnostic accuracy of the anxiety and depression detector. Gen Hosp Psychiatry 2006;28(2):108–118. www.sciencedirect.com/science?_obArticleURL&_udi=B6T70–4TCCCXY-5&_user=10&_handle=V-WA-AW-AD-MsSA.
6. Othmer E, Othmer SC, Othmer JP. Psychiatric interview, history, and mental status examination. In: Sadock BJ, Sadock VA, eds. Kaplan and Sadock's Comprehensive Textbook of Psychiatry, 8th ed., vol. 1. Philadelphia: Lippincott Williams & Wilkins, 2005:815–816.
7. National Center for Posttraumatic Stress Disorder. Screening for PTSD in a primary care setting. http://www.ncptsd.va.gov/facts/disasters/fs_screen_disaster.html.
8. Scheiber SC. The psychiatric interview, history, and mental status examination. In: Hales RE, Yudofsky SC, eds.Textbook of Clinical Psychiatry, 4th ed. Washington, DC: American Psychiatric Publishing, 2003:155–187.
9. Shader, RI. The mental status examination. In: Shader RI. ed. Manual of Psychiatric Therapeutics, 3rd ed. Philadelphia: Lippincott Williams & Wilkins, 2003: 9–16.
10. Blacker D. Psychiatric rating scales. In: Sadock BJ, Sadock VA,eds. Kaplan and Sadock's Comprehensive Textbook of Psychiatry, 8th ed., vol. 1. Philadelphia: Lippincott Williams & Wilkins, 2005: 945–947.
11. Freeston MH, Landouceur R, Thibodeau N, Gagnon F, Rheaume J. The Beck Anxiety Inventory. Psychometric properties of a French translation. Encephale 1994;20(abstr). www.ncbi.nlm.nih.gov/entrez/query.fcgi?cmd=Retrieve&db=PubMed&list_uids=81.
12. Beck Anxiety Inventory. http://www.cps.nova.edu/~cpphelp/BAI.html.
13. Connor KM, Davidson JRT, Churchill LE, Sherwood A, Weisler RH. Psychometric properties of the social phobia inventory. Br J Psychiatry 2000;176:379–386. bjp.rcpsych.org/cgi/content/full/176/4/379.
14. Liebowitz MR. Social phobia. Mod Probl Pharmacopsychiatry 1987;22:141–173.

3
Psychopharmacology

John R. Vanin

Psychopharmacology is defined as the science of drugs having an effect on psychomotor behavior and emotional states [1]. The primary care practitioner has an opportunity to apply skillful pharmacologic practices to safely and effectively manage patients with anxiety disorders and their coexisting problems. Having a good grasp of psychiatric principles, medicine, and pharmacology allows the primary care clinician to comfortably use the various classes of medications commonly used to treat anxiety disorders. These medications include antidepressants, which are among the most effective antianxiety agents. Most antidepressants are broadly effective for many types of disorders. The selective serotonin reuptake inhibitors (SSRIs) have become a mainstay for the treatment of anxiety disorders [2]. Other categories of medications for the treatment of anxiety disorders, used alone or as adjunctive therapies, include the benzodiazepines, azapirones, β-adrenergic receptor blockers, antihistamines, anticonvulsants, and antipsychotic medications [2,3]. These categories of medications are discussed in more detail in this chapter, along with a brief discussion of novel antianxiety therapeutics.

Appropriate pharmacotherapy of anxiety disorders relies on various aspects of psychopharmacology, many of which apply to the treatment of other medical disorders. The art and science of psychopharmacology considers many areas including appropriate diagnosis, determining symptoms that are medication responsive (target symptoms), and a patient who is well informed about his/her illness and the treatment plan [2,4,5]. It is very important to keep in mind that comorbidity is extremely common when evaluating and treating anxiety disorders. Table 1.5 in Chapter 1 lists several principles of psychopharmacology for the primary care clinician that can be helpful in daily practice.

The therapeutic alliance relies heavily on a clinician who listens, educates, and collaborates, and does not dictate. This certainly applies to the area of basic psychopharmacology. Early efficacy with the antianxiety medication, improved functioning, as well as minimal side effects also facilitate compliance and a good long-term outcome [5]. For most patients with anxiety disorders, pharmacotherapy or empirically proven psychotherapy such as cognitive-behavioral therapy, or a combination approach, is an appropriate treatment option [2]. Relieving symptoms and improving function equates with improvement in quality of life.

NEUROTRANSMITTERS

To improve one's grasp of basic psychopharmacology and how effective psychiatric medications exert their beneficial as well as side effects, this chapter provides an overview of neurotransmitters (chemical messengers), receptors, and other biological information. The information includes general principles and definitions that can facilitate a better understanding of anxiety disorders and their comorbidities.

The basic definition of a neurotransmitter is a substance that excites or inhibits a target cell [1]. A more detailed and technical classic definition of a neurotransmitter includes the following criteria [6]:

- Synthesized and released from neurons
- Released from nerve terminals in an identifiable form (chemical or pharmacological)
- Interacts with a postsynaptic receptor with the same effects seen with presynaptic neuron stimulation
- Interacts with a postsynaptic receptor with a specific pharmacology
- Terminates actions by an active process

Under certain circumstances, some neurotransmitters, neuro-modulators, and neurohormones do not meet all the criteria [6], but are still referred to as such.

Compounds that are active in the central nervous system (CNS) are either made locally in the brain or cross the blood–brain barrier. Dozens of substances within the CNS function as neuro-transmitters. Different chemicals can convey different information within the brain. It is interesting to note that a single neuron can distinguish information from many different incoming nerve terminals by possessing different receptor sites. The same chemical can convey different messages as well, depending on its action on receptor subtypes [6]. Other important ways of conveying information in the brain include different neuronal firing patterns and spatial coding [6].

RECEPTORS

Receptors recognize specific molecules such as neurotransmitters and hormones, and this process results in activation. This process may be pictured as several dominos standing in a row; tapping the first one forward sets the others in motion. A typical cellular response in neurons includes voltage changes across a membrane that result in changes in neuronal excitability [6]. There are four groups of transmembrane signaling systems, and a brief description of these is listed in Table 3.1 [6]. These are very important concepts for our current understanding of neurotransmission.

More than 80% of all known receptors in the body are G-protein–coupled receptors [6]. G proteins were named because of their binding ability to guanine nucleotides [6]. Autoreceptors are common to this group. The autoreceptors that help regulate neuronal firing rates are called somatodendritic autoreceptors. Those that regulate the amount of neurotransmitter released are called nerve terminal autoreceptors. G-protein–coupled receptors are also regulated by other processes [6], including the following:

- Desensitization (cells rapidly adapt to stimulation)
- Downregulation (prolonged or repeated activation leads to reduced number of receptors)
- Trafficking (lessens signaling by rapidly and reversibly removing receptors)

SEROTONERGIC SYSTEM

Serotonin is also known as 5-hydroxytryptamine (5-HT). Serotonin was named because of its activity as a vasoconstrictor in the blood. Two percent of the body's serotonin is located in the brain, where the highest concentration is in the raphe nuclei of the brainstem [7]. The neurons project widely throughout the CNS. Serotonin is

---

TABLE 3.1. Transmembrane signaling systems

- Inotropic: transmembrane ion fluxes—very rapid response (e.g., glutamate, GABA)
- G-protein–coupled response: intracellular second messengers—slower response (e.g., catecholamines, serotonin, acetylcholine, various peptides, sensory signals)
- Receptor tyrosine kinases: acute synaptic function changes—long-term effect on neuronal growth and survival; intrinsic enzymatic activity (e.g., neurotropic factors, cytokines)
- Nuclear receptors: directly regulate transcription after activation by lipophilic molecules (e.g., hormones)

Adapted from ref. [6].

a principal neurotransmitter that is involved in the regulation of many biological functions including anxiety, mood, sleep, appetite, memory, cognition, and sexual behavior [8].

Neurons in the brain synthesize serotonin. The amino acid tryptophan is hydroxylated by the enzyme tryptophan hydroxylase, forming 5-hydroxytryptophan. This is then decarboxylated to 5-hydroxytryptamine, or serotonin [7]. The precursor tryptophan comes primarily from diet, and it crosses the blood–brain barrier. The enzyme tryptophan hydroxylase is the rate-limiting step in serotonin synthesis. Termination of serotonin effects in the synaptic cleft occurs by way of the 5-HT transporter. 5-Hydroxytryptamine is taken up into the presynaptic terminals and goes back into storage vesicles or is metabolized.

Medications such as SSRIs and many tricyclic antidepressants (TCAs) bind to the transporter and block the reuptake of 5-HT. This leads to an increase in 5-HT levels in the synapse and starts a cascade of effects downstream. The SSRIs and serotonin (5-HT) bind to the same transporter site [6].

SEROTONIN RECEPTORS

At least 14 serotonin (5-HT) receptors and subtypes have been identified. All are G-protein–coupled receptors, except for 5-HT3, which is inotropic or a ligand-gated ion channel [6,7,9]. Serotonin can both cause and relieve anxiety, depending on the area of the brain and the receptor subtype involved. 5-HT2A receptors mediate most anxiety producing effects, and 5-HT1A receptors are involved in antianxiety effects and perhaps adaptive responses [9]. Table 3.2 lists the 5-HT receptors, including subtypes, and

TABLE 3.2. Serotonin (5-HT) receptors and subtypes

5-HT1 receptor
* 5-HT1A, B, D, E, F
5-HT1A—clinical relevance includes anxiolytic effect
5-HT2 receptor
* 5-HT2A, B, C
5-HT2C—clinical relevance includes regulation of anxiety
5-HT3 receptor
5-HT4 receptor—clinical relevance includes modulation of anxiety
5-HT5 receptor
* 5-HT alpha, beta
5-HT6 receptor
5-HT7 receptor—possible regulation of circadian rhythms; acute stress may alter expression

Adapted from refs. [6], [7], and [10].

gives examples of their relevance to anxiety [6,7,10]. Indeed, 5-HT dysregulation has been identified as playing a role in the pathogenesis of psychiatric disorders including anxiety disorders, and medications that improve serotonin transmission can effectively treat these disorders [9].

NORADRENERGIC SYSTEM

Norepinephrine (noradrenaline) is produced from the amino acid precursor tyrosine. Tyrosine yields L-dopa by way of the enzyme tyrosine hydroxylase, which is the rate-limiting enzyme [7]. L-dopa is converted to dopamine by dopa decarboxylase. The enzyme dopamine β-hydroxylase converts dopamine to norepinephrine. The noradrenergic cell groups in the brain are located in the locus ceruleus and the lateral tegmental nuclei of the brainstem [6,7,10]. Both project extensively, and the locus ceruleus, which probably plays a modulation and integrative role, is the most widely projecting nucleus in the CNS [6].

Norepinephrine neurotransmission is terminated by the action of the norepinephrine transporter protein. Norepinephrine is transported from the synaptic cleft back into the neuron. Adrenergic receptors include α and β groups with several subtypes (Table 3.3) [6,7,10,11]. Norepinephrine receptors belong to the G-protein family. These receptors are found in the CNS as well as peripherally [11].

DOPAMINERGIC SYSTEM

Dopamine is a precursor of norepinephrine and epinephrine. Tyrosine crosses the blood–brain barrier into brain cells, and the enzyme tyrosine hydroxylase converts this amino acid to L-dihydroxyphenylalanine (L-dopa). This conversion is the rate-limiting

---

TABLE 3.3. Adrenergic receptors and subtypes

Alpha 1A, B, D
 • Activation of α-1 receptors may stimulate activity of serotonin neurons
Alpha 2A/D, B, C
 • Alpha-2A-stimulation inhibits firing of locus ceruleus neurons; stimulation of α-2 receptors reduces sympathetic and augments parasympathetic nervous system activity; activation of α-2 receptors may inhibit serotonin neurons
Beta-1—major role in regulation of heart function
Beta-2—role in bronchial muscle relaxation
Beta-3

Adapted from refs. [6], [7], [10], and [11].

step for dopamine synthesis [7]. Dopamine is formed by the decarboxylation of L-dopa by the enzyme L-aromatic amino acid decarboxylase. Termination of the dopamine signal in the synapse occurs primarily via reuptake by the dopamine transporter into the presynaptic terminal [6,7]. After reuptake, the neurotransmitter is either degraded or taken up into vesicles. The enzymes that degrade dopamine include monoamine oxidase (MAO) and catechol-o-methyltransferase (COMT). Monoamine oxidase B preferentially deaminates dopamine [10]. Homovanillic acid is the predominant metabolite of dopamine in humans.

The majority of the dopamine cells are located in the anterior midbrain, and the projections include the striatum, cerebral cortex, and other subcortical structures [7]. Dopamine receptors belong to the G-protein–coupled receptor class [7]. The dopamine receptors include two general classes and several subtypes:

- D1—includes D1 and D5
- D2—includes D2, D3, D4

CHOLINERGIC SYSTEM

Acetylcholine (Ach) is synthesized from acetyl coenzyme A and choline via the enzyme choline acetyltransferase [6,7]. Most of the choline is transported into the brain from the bloodstream. The rate-limiting step in Ach synthesis is the active transport of choline into the neurons in the brain [10]. Ach is stored in synaptic vesicles, and after release, the signal is terminated primarily by the enzyme acetylcholinesterase [7]. The acetylcholine is rapidly degraded by hydrolysis, and choline is taken back up into the presynaptic terminal. A second class of cholinesterase enzymes involving butyrylcholinesterase is located in the glia as well as other areas in the body [10]. There are several cholinergic pathways in the CNS. Some act as local circuit neurons (interneurons) and others project to connect different brain regions [6,7]. Acetylcholine-containing neurons are located in several CNS areas including the basal forebrain complex, pontomesencephalotegmental complex, and striatum.

Cholinergic receptors consist of two major types with several subtypes. These include muscarinic receptors, which are G-protein coupled and linked to second messenger systems in the cortex, hippocampus, amygdala, thalamus, and other subcortical structures, as well as nicotinic receptors, which act on sodium channels (inotropic) [6,7]. Muscarinic and nicotinic receptors and subtypes are listed in Table 3.4 [6, 7].

TABLE 3.4. Cholinergic receptors and subtypes

* Muscarinic—M1, M2, M3, M4, M5
* Nicotinic—alpha (7 forms); beta (3 forms)

Adapted from refs. [6] and [7].

GABAERGIC SYSTEM

γ-Aminobutyric acid (GABA) is the major inhibitory neurotransmitter in the CNS, but it can produce an excitatory effect at times [6,12,13]. It is found in high concentration throughout the brain. Nonpyramidal cortical neurons as well as other CNS areas such as the thalamus and basal ganglia utilize GABA [6]. To produce GABA, glucose is converted to α-ketoglutarate in the axon terminals, which is then transaminated to glutamate by GABA α-oxoglutarate transaminase. Glutamate is decarboxylated by glutamic acid decarboxylase to form GABA [6,7]. The rate-limiting enzyme is glutamic acid decarboxylase. γ-Aminobutyric acid can react with many presynaptic and postsynaptic receptors after release by the presynaptic terminal. Catabolism of GABA yields succinic acid via the action of GABA α-oxoglutarate transaminase (which is also involved in synthesis) and then α-ketoglutarate, which can then be used to make more GABA [6]. The effects of GABA are terminated in the synapse by reuptake via GABA transporters.

There are two major types of GABA receptors: GABA-A and GABA-B. There are five subunit classes of GABA-A (alpha, beta, gamma, delta, and epsilon) and at least 18 further subtypes [6,12].

γ-Aminobutyric acid A is the most prevalent type in the mammalian CNS and it contains a very important transmembrane chloride channel. When activated, this channel opens, resulting in hyperpolarization, which suppresses neuron excitability. Benzodiazepines, as an example, bind to a site on GABA-A, leading to opening of the chloride channel and an inhibitory response.

GLUTAMATERGIC SYSTEM

Glutamate is an excitatory amino acid. It cannot penetrate the blood–brain barrier and so must be produced in the brain. Glutamate is present in high concentrations in the brain [6]. The major proportion of glutamate comes from glucose and the transamination of α-ketoglutarate, but a small amount is formed from glutamine [6,7]. The synthetic and metabolic enzymes are located in neurons and glial cells. There are several major transporter proteins. The glutamate transporter, located on the presynaptic axon terminal, terminates the action of glutamate by reuptake [7]. Phosphorylation

TABLE 3.5. Glutamate receptors and subtypes

Inotropic
- *N*-methyl-D-aspartate (NMDA)
- Alpha-amino-3-hydroxy-5-methyl-4-isoxazole propionic acid (AMPA)
- Kainate

Metabotropic
- 8 types; 3 subgroups (I, II, III)

Adapted from ref. [7].

by protein kinases may differentially regulate glutamate transporters and glutamate uptake, but this activity is not well understood [6]. It is interesting to note that glutamate is a precursor for most of the GABA that is made in the neurons [13].

There are two major subtypes of glutamate receptors. Inotropic receptors are ion channels within the neuronal membrane. Metabotropic receptors are G-protein–coupled receptors. Table 3.5 lists these receptors as well as several other subtypes of glutamate receptors [7].

NEUROPEPTIDES

Neuropeptides modulate the classical neurotransmitters [7]. They are first synthesized as a precursor protein and stored in large vesicles [6]. Higher frequencies stimulate the release of neuropeptides from neurons [6]. A common clinical example of the action of neuropeptides includes corticotropin-releasing factor (CRF) hormone secreted by the hypothalamus stimulating the pituitary release of adrenocorticotropic hormone (ACTH), which results in cortisol production by the adrenal gland. Table 3.6 lists examples of peptides that may be relevant to anxiety disorders [6,8].

TABLE 3.6. Peptides that may be relevant to anxiety disorders

- Corticotropin-releasing factor (CRF) (implicated in anxiety symptoms)
- Adrenocorticotropic hormone (ACTH) (dysregulated in mood disorders)
- Thyrotropin-releasing factor (TRF) (potential antidepressant effects)
- Cholecystokinin (CCK) (anxiety, panic)
- Substance P (member of tachykinin neuropeptide family; may alleviate anxiety)
- Neuropeptide Y (potential endogenous anxiolytic)
- Vasopressin (potential novel anxiolytics)
- Opioid/related peptides (possible antidepressant activity)

Adapted from refs. [6] and [8].

PHARMACOKINETICS AND PHARMACODYNAMICS

Pharmacokinetics may be defined as the study of metabolism and action of drugs [1]. When a patient uses a medication, several phases of pharmacokinetics occur: absorption, distribution, metabolism, and elimination [14,15]. Pharmacodynamics is defined as the study of drugs and their actions [1]. Patients are different in many ways and the dose of medication and the pharmacological effect can vary for many reasons including gender, age, and organ function (Table 3.7) [14]. Understanding the general principles of pharmacokinetics and pharmacodynamics enables the practitioner to rationally individualize dosages. It is important to keep in mind that the body acts on medications in certain ways, and medications, in turn, act on the body.

The desired therapeutic goal requires the clinician to use a rational approach regarding the drug dosage regimen, and this approach is based on scientific principles and clinical experience. The pharmacological response from medications differs widely among patients regarding the dose of medications and the frequency of dosing [14]. The primary care practitioner wants to avoid underdosing and an unsatisfactory response, but also must monitor for overdosing that may result in toxicity. A common clinical error is the treatment of specific symptoms instead of treating the underlying disorder or syndrome. Sometimes this may seem like the right clinical approach at the time, and at other times this approach may be secondary to frustration. For example, a patient with an anxiety disorder such as generalized anxiety

TABLE 3.7. Factors affecting variability of medication doses and effects

- Physiology
- Age
- Gender
- Culture
- Illness/severity
- Comorbidity
- Drug metabolizing enzymes
- Renal function
- GI function/food
- Concomitant use of other drugs/interactions
- Active metabolites
- Pharmacogenetics (study of the genetic basis for differences in drug effects)

Adapted from ref. [14].

may suffer from nervousness, sleep difficulty, nonspecific somatic symptoms such as pain, and gastrointestinal complaints. A common potential error is initially to treat various symptoms with too many medications, including a low-dose antidepressant (that may be maintained at a subtherapeutic dose), a benzodiazepine, a separate sleep medication, an analgesic for pain, and perhaps something for the functional gastrointestinal symptoms. This regimen is not necessarily wrong, but one should consider starting with a low-dose antidepressant and titrating upward as tolerated to a therapeutic dose. Adding a benzodiazepine to help control the anxiety initially and as a sleep aid would also be acceptable. The pain and gastrointestinal concerns may thus be alleviated with fewer medications, at least at this stage of treatment. Utilizing patient education and psychotherapeutic techniques would help the patient understand the anxiety disorder and maintain better compliance with the management plan. As the syndrome of generalized anxiety disorder is controlled, the pain, insomnia, and gastrointestinal symptoms often disappear and other medications may not be necessary. On the other hand, many patients have psychiatric conditions that require concomitant use of several psychotropics, and this use, based on sound pharmacological principles, is called rational polypharmacy [4].

Drug interactions occur when another drug or substance alters the pharmacological action of a medication [4]. Polypharmacy is common in clinical practice, and the practitioner must be alert for potential drug interactions. Understanding an important drug metabolizing system called the cytochrome P-450 (CYP) enzyme system enables the primary care practitioner to recognize and even predict many drug–drug interactions. Three types of drug interactions include pharmacokinetic, pharmacodynamic, and idiosyncratic interactions [4]. Despite the prevalence of clinical polypharmacy, noninteraction of medications is far more common than interactions [16]. On the other hand, some clinicians feel many drug–drug interactions are clinically relevant and underestimated.

PHARMACOKINETICS

Drug concentration changes in the plasma over time are an important aspect of pharmacokinetics, and the measurement of these concentrations can be clinically useful. Plasma drug levels can be very useful for safe and effective adjustments for many medications such as lithium, some anticonvulsants, and tricyclic antidepressants [14]. Plasma drug concentrations are not routinely monitored for most of the medications commonly used to treat anxiety disorders, such as the SSRIs and benzodiazepines.

Population pharmacokinetics provides estimates of drug and metabolite half-lives, which can help predict washout times after a drug is discontinued [14]. This type of information can be clinically useful to the primary care practitioner when switching among the antidepressants and other antianxiety medications.

Absorption

The route of administration is a major factor regarding a medication's onset and duration of action. Absorption is not a consideration when a medication is given intravenously [16] because the drug reaches the systemic circulation immediately after administration. Intramuscular (IM) administration is also generally rapid, but absorption of some medications is slow and erratic [14]. For example, IM injection of chlordiazepoxide (Librium) may yield incomplete bioavailability, while IM administration of lorazepam (Ativan) and diazepam (Valium) results in essentially complete systemic absorption [14,16].

Access to the systemic circulation is more complex after oral administration. The main route of administration of psychopharmacological medications for anxiety disorders is the oral route. Most psychoactive medications are highly lipophilic (an affinity for fat) and generally absorbed well in the first part of small intestine. The efficiency of absorption by the oral route, and thus the onset of clinical action, is determined by many factors including the patient's physiological state, the medication formulation, and the timing of administration around meals [14]. Most medications are best absorbed on an empty stomach because the presence of food or other substances such as antacids decreases the rate of absorption. Some medications can be given with or without food, and in some cases the administration of a medication with food increases plasma concentration of the medication. A possible explanation for this is that the food-induced increase in hepatic blood flow allows more unabsorbed drug to escape first-pass hepatic uptake and metabolism [14].

The absolute systemic availability (bioavailability) of a medication is the portion of a drug absorbed from the site of administration [15,16]. The bioavailability of a medication administered orally is the fraction of the dose that reaches the systemic circulation [16]. Mathematically, possible values range from 0 (no detectable oral amount reaches the systemic circulation) to 1 (entire oral dose reaches systemic circulation) [16].

Many psychotropics have incomplete bioavailability for several reasons, which include poor absorption and presystemic extraction (metabolism by the gastrointestinal mucosa or the liver) [14,16]. After oral absorption, the medication enters the portal circulation and enters the liver. It can undergo extensive metabolism in the liver cells before it reaches the systemic circulation. This is called the first-pass effect or first-pass metabolism. The first-pass effect may decrease the amount of parent drug and increase the quantity of metabolites. After first-pass metabolism, some metabolites are excreted into the bile and subsequently the small bowel. The lipid-soluble metabolites are reabsorbed into the portal circulation and then the systemic circulation. The metabolites may be pharmacologically similar or different from the parent drug and may be active. The first-pass effect is a major source of pharmacokinetic variability [14]. Clinicians must keep in mind that some medical conditions, as well as coadministering medications, can affect first-pass effects and the resultant medication effects. Common factors affecting bioavailability are listed in Table 3.8 [15].

Presystemic metabolism of medications often occurs as the result of action by CYP enzymes, located in the luminal epithelium of the small intestine as well as in the liver [14]. The enzymes primarily involved in drug metabolism include CYP1A2, CYP2C, CYP2D6, and CYP3A3/4 [4]. The CYP enzymes are responsible for most human drug metabolism [16]. Although located in many areas in the body, the enzymes in the intestine and liver are the most important regarding drug availability and clearance. Many useful psychopharmacological medications are substrates (metabolized by a given enzyme) of 3A4. Approximately 70% of total CYP in the human intestine is represented by 3A4 [14]. The liver contains much larger amounts of the CYP3A protein than does the small intestine, but the intestine has a considerable effect on presystemic medication metabolism [14]. Table 3.9 lists examples of substrates, inhibitors, and inducers of liver CYPs involved in drug metabolism [4,14,16].

The transmembrane transport pump P-glycoprotein (P-gp) may also be involved in drug interactions [14]. This is also known as the multidrug resistance protein.

Most psychotropic drugs that are ultimately available in the systemic circulation are highly lipophilic and readily pass the

TABLE 3.8. Common factors influencing medication bioavailability

- Physicochemical properties
- Formulation
- Disease states influencing gastrointestinal function or first-pass effect
- Precipitation of drug at injection site

Adapted from ref. [15].

TABLE 3.9. Examples of substrates, inhibitors, and inducers of cytochrome P-450 (CYP) enzymes involved in drug metabolism

CYP1A2

Substrates

Aminophylline	Haloperidol +	Phenacetin	Verapamil +
Amitriptyline	Imipramine +	Propranolol	Warfarin +
Caffeine +	Methadone	Tacrine	
Clozapine	Olanzapine	Theophylline +	

Inhibitors

Cimetidine	Grapefruit juice
Enoxacin	Ketoconazole
Fluoroquinolones (ciprofloxacin, norfloxacin)	

Inducers

Charcoal-broiled beef
Cigarette smoke   Omeprazole
Cruciferous vegetables
Marijuana smoke

CYP2C9/10

Substrates

Amitriptyline +	Diclofenac	Propranolol +	Tolbutamide
Metoclopramide	Phenytoin	Tetrahydro-cannabinol +	Warfarin +

Inhibitors

Cimetidine	Fluoxetine	Modafinil
Disulfiram	Fluvoxamine	Ritonavir
Fluconazole	D-propoxyphene	Sulfaphenazole

Inducers

Phenytoin	Rifampin	Secobarbital

CYP2C19

Substrates

Amitriptyline +	Desmethyl-diazepam +	Imipramine +	Omeprazole +
Barbiturates	Diazepam +	S-mephenytoin	Piroxicam
Citalopram +	Divalproex	Moclobemide	Tenoxicam
Clomipramine +	Ibuprofen	Naproxen	

Inhibitors

Fluoxetine	Fluvoxamine	Omeprazole

Inducers

Rifampin

Continued

TABLE 3.9. *Continued*

CYP2D6			

Substrates

Most antipsychotics (includes haloperidol +, risperidone, thioridazine)

Amitriptyline +	Flecainide	Ondansetron +	Trazodone
Citalopram +	Fluoxetine +	Orphenadrine	Type IC antiarrhythmics
Codeine +	Galanthamine	Paroxetine	
Debrisoquin	Imipramine +	Pindolol	Venlafaxine +
Desipramine	Metoclopramide	Propafenone	
Dextromethorphan	Metoprolol	Propranolol +	
Donepezil	Mexiletine	Timolol	
Encainide	Nortriptyline	Tramadol	

Inhibitors

Bupropion	Fluoxetine	Quinidine	Terbinafine
Cimetidine	Paroxetine	Ritonavir	
Diphenhydramine	Phenothiazines	Sertraline	

Inducers

None documented in vivo

CPY3A 3/4/5			

Substrates

Acetaminophen	Cyclosporine	Loratadine	Rifampin
Alprazolam	Dapsone +	Lovastatin	Sertraline
Amiodarone	Desmethyl-diazepam +	Midazolam	Statins
Amitriptyline +	Diltiazem	Nefazodone	Steroids
Astemizole	Donepezil	Nicardipine	Tamoxifen
Bupropion	Erythromycin	Nifedipine	Terfenadine
Caffeine +	Estradiol	Omeprazole +	Testosterone
Calcium channel blockers	Ethinylestradiol	Ondansetron	Trazodone
Carbamazepine	Ethosuximide	Orphenadrine	Triazolam
Cisapride	Fluoxetine	Oxcarbazepine	Venlafaxine +
Citalopram +	Galanthamine	Pimozide	Verapamil +
Clarithromycin	Haloperidol +	Progesterone	Zolpidem +
Clonazepam	Imipramine +	Propafenone	
Clozapine +	Lamotrigine	Quetiapine	
Codeine +	Lidocaine	Quinidine	

Inhibitors

Cimetidine	Fluoxetine	Itraconazole	Saquinavir
Clarithromycin	Fluvoxamine	Ketoconazole	Sertraline (weak)
Diltiazem	Grapefruit juice (naringin)	Nefazodone	Verapamil
Erythromycin	Indinavir	Ritonavir	

Continued

TABLE 3.9. *Continued*

Inducers

Barbiturates	Dexamethasone	Rifampin
Carbamazepine	Phenytoin	St. John's Wort

CYP2A6

Substrates

Coumarin	Nicotine

Inhibitors
Tranylcypromine

Inducers
Barbiturates

2B6

Substrates

Bupropion	Tamoxifen	Cyclophosphamide
Nicotine	Diazepam +	

Inducers
Phenobarbital
Cyclophosphamide (in vitro)

P4502E1

Substrates

Caffeine +	Dapsone +	Ethanol

Inhibitors
Disulfiram

Inducers
Ethanol

Adapted from refs. [4], [14], and [16].
+More than one enzyme known to be involved in metabolism.

TABLE 3.10. Common shared features
of most psychotropics

- Lipophilic
- Availability to the brain
- Rapid absorption
- Complete absorption
- High first-pass effect
- Large volume of distribution

Adapted from ref. [15].

blood–brain barrier into the CNS. Psychotropics, being highly lipophilic, share several features (Table 3.10) [15].

Physicochemical properties of a medication play an important role in the absorption from the gastrointestinal tract and the penetration into the brain. Polarity is one such property. The more polar a medication, the slower the absorption from the gastrointestinal (GI) tract into the systemic circulation and the slower the penetration into the brain [15]. For example, the most polar benzodiazepine oxazepam is a poor sedative because it is slowly absorbed into the systemic circulation as well as into the brain. Lorazepam, a less polar compound, is rapidly absorbed and penetrates into the brain rapidly [15].

Other physicochemical properties of a drug include peak concentrations (C_{max}) and time to peak concentration (T_{max}). The C_{max} will generally be inversely related to the T_{max} [15]; namely, the shorter the time for drug absorption, the higher the peak concentration.

Fast absorption may not always be desirable, however, and the practitioner must be aware of potential drug toxicity related to C_{max} [15]. At times, changing a formulation of the medication and dividing the dose into smaller amounts and administering the medication more frequently is a safer approach. The amounts of medication absorbed and average concentrations in the plasma will be the same, but the peak concentration will be lower and the trough concentration higher. This could result in greater tolerability and safety for the patient.

Formulation factors are extremely important with regard to obtaining plasma minimum effective concentrations. Generally, the dosage formulations ranging from most rapid to slowest rate of drug release orally are solutions, suspensions, tablets, enteric-coated tablets, and capsules [14]. Medications with short elimination half-lives may be formulated into sustained or slow-release tablets or capsules. These can be effective when given once or twice a day (instead of multiple times per day), which can positively affect adverse effects and patient compliance. It is important to recognize that regardless of dosage formulation, the drug elimination rate is unaffected by the rate or extent of absorption [14].

Generic formulations of psychotropics are becoming more available. According to the U.S. Food and Drug Administration, a generic medication is comparable to a brand name medication if there is no more than an approximate 20% variation either way (±20%) in bioavailability [15]. It is important for the clinician to recognize that there can theoretically be an approximate 40% total bioavailability difference between two generic preparations of the same medication. It should also be noted that some patients complain that they are intolerant or "allergic" to some component of generic preparations of the same drug made by one manufacturer versus another.

Distribution

Distribution of a medication to the organs occurs in direct proportion to the fat and protein content after the medication is in the systemic circulation. The rate of distribution depends on several factors including membrane permeability, vascularity, and hydration state [14,15]. The highly lipid-soluble medications accumulate in the brain to the same extent that they accumulate in adipose tissue, but the rate of accumulation in the brain is much faster than in adipose tissue [15].

When a single dose of a medication is given, the drug reaches a peak concentration and then drops primarily due to drug distribution, rather than elimination. Drugs are distributed to various body compartments including fat, water, brain, and bone. The volume of distribution describes how widely a drug is distributed in the body. The rate of drug distribution to the various organs depends on several factors, including lipid solubility, ionizability, and binding affinity for plasma proteins and tissue [14,15]. A very important concept to recognize is that only free or unbound drug can distribute between plasma and tissues to produce a behavioral response. This is generally a small amount, because most psychotropics are highly protein bound (more than 90% of the total plasma concentration) [15]. The "second-dose effect" [14] may occur with the ingestion of substances such as caffeine. When a second drug dose is taken immediately after the cessation of the first dose effects, the intensity and duration of the second dose effects may be greater and longer than those of the first dose. When the second drug dose is given before the previous dose has been eliminated, the second and subsequent doses produce a greater effect than the initial dose, but the relative intensity diminishes with subsequent doses.

Drug concentrations can vary widely among tissues, but eventually equilibrium occurs between concentrations in plasma and tissue [14]. The concentration of a drug in brain tissue may be quite different from its plasma concentration. The minimal effective concentration of a drug determined from the plasma may reflect a minimal effective concentration in brain tissue or other organs [14]. It should also be noted that drug binding must be measured using mathematical models, since binding in tissues cannot be directly measured.

Displacement of a bound drug from plasma proteins may result from drug–drug interactions. More unbound drug could thus be available to interact with receptors, which could cause beneficial or detrimental effects. It is important to be aware of this possibility, but there are few documented cases of psychoactive drugs

causing significant clinical consequences because of displacement
[14]. The body seems to be very efficient in handling drug-binding
interactions.

Metabolism

Most psychotropics undergo hepatic biotransformation, involving
one or several of the following steps [15]:

- Hydroxylation
- Demethylation
- Oxidation
- Sulfoxide formation

The basic purpose of drug metabolism is to form more polar
metabolites (water soluble), which are more readily excreted in the
urine or bile. Most drugs are extensively biotransformed prior to
elimination, but some undergo simple conjugation with glucuronic
acid [15], which can occur in most organs, not just the liver. Other
medications are excreted unmetabolized.

Some drugs induce the metabolism of other drugs as well
as themselves (autoinduction). Other drugs inhibit specific liver
enzymes. The rate of drug conversion depends on the rate of delivery
to the liver, which is determined by arterial flow [15]. After
a drug enters the systemic circulation, cardiac left ventricular
function delivers blood back to the liver. Diseases that directly
or indirectly affect liver function such as liver disease, metabolic
disorders, and cardiac disease can affect medication metabolism
[15]. For example, beta-blockers decrease arterial flow and may
slow the metabolism of medications that undergo extensive liver
biotransformation.

Elimination

Psychotropic drugs are eliminated or cleared from the body by
kidney excretion and biotransformation. The kidney clearance of a
medication is either unchanged or conjugated, and biotransformation
involves a change to polar metabolites (more water and less
lipid soluble compounds) primarily by the liver [14]. Clearance may
be defined as the volume of fluid from which a drug is irreversibly
removed per unit of time [14]. Drug extraction from the blood is
rarely 100% [14]. Plasma protein binding can restrict drug extraction
by an organ. Also, some drugs can escape the presystemic elimination
process and go into the systemic circulation intact [14].

Another clearance concept that must be recognized and understood
is the elimination half-life. The elimination half-life is the

time required for the plasma concentration of a drug to decline by 50%, assuming distribution has reached equilibrium [16]. Clearance and volume of distribution determine the elimination half-life [16].

MULTIPLE DOSING AND STEADY STATE

In the treatment of mental disorders, including the anxiety disorders, pharmacotherapy is usually required on a repeated basis. The second and subsequent doses are usually given before the initial dose is completely eliminated, and this results in drug accumulation [14]. Linear or first-order kinetics is defined as the amount of drug eliminated per unit time and is directly proportional to its plasma concentration [14,15]. Accumulation does not occur indefinitely. A steady state occurs when the amount of drug entering the body is equal to the amount of drug leaving the body [14]. The total concentration of a drug in the plasma at steady state will not change as long as the dose and the dose schedule stays unchanged or other factors do not alter the metabolism or elimination rate [15]. For example, after a period of continuous dosing of a medication, the body retains a portion from several doses and an equivalent amount of medication eliminated is replaced by an equivalent amount of administered medication. A steady state requires approximately four to five elimination half-lives from the point of initial administration of a medication, and the same amount of time is required for a new steady state to be achieved after an increase or decrease in daily dose or for a wash-out of the medication after discontinuation [14]. In other words, the longer the half-life of a medication, the longer the period of time to achieve steady state or elimination from the body after discontinuation. The rate at which a medication is washed out of the body can be very important clinically. Toxic effects can be reversed much more quickly if a medication has a short half-life. However, longer half-life medications tend to exhibit less rebound and withdrawal symptoms than medications with shorter half-lives. A true steady state occurs only with a constant-rate intravenous administration of a drug [14], but clinically we speak of an average steady-state concentration occurring between the dosage interval peak and trough concentrations [14].

Zero-order kinetics occurs when only a fixed amount of drug is eliminated per unit time regardless of plasma concentration [15]. The enzymes for biotransformation and elimination are saturated. First-order kinetics occurs when the amount of drug eliminated per unit time is directly proportional to its plasma concentration [15]. There is a linear relationship between change of dose and change of plasma level. When practitioners prescribe additional medication with zero-order kinetics, they must be aware that medication levels will be higher but they will not know how much higher.

Another interesting pharmacokinetic concept is linearity. Linearity is defined as maintaining a stable clearance across the usual dosage range [14]. The size of a dosage increase results in a proportional change in steady-state concentration within the linear dose range [14]. A patient may require an increase in dose, but giving the dose once a day may not be tolerated. Doubling the daily dose of a medication may result in an adequate average steady-state concentration, but there is an increased risk of toxicity or inadequate concentration because of the change in the peak and trough levels with a once- or twice-a-day regimen. Clinically, one could increase the total daily dose and divide it into more frequent dosing. This allows for a reduction of the peak and trough concentrations and keeps the average steady-state concentration in the desired range. This perhaps would allow the medication to be better tolerated.

The minimum requirement for a drug's onset and offset of action is determined by pharmacokinetics [15]. Pharmacokinetics determines how frequently medications must be taken for the desired therapeutic effect as well as how long the medication's action will persist. The safe and effective use of medication combinations requires knowledge about pharmacokinetic interactions. Changes with aging or disease can alter the pharmacokinetics of a medication [15]. The elderly, for example, may have a decrease in intracellular water, protein binding, and tissue mass, as well as an increase in total body fat. They may also have a decrease in intestinal absorption, increase in gastric pH, increase in free-drug fraction, decrease in metabolism, and a decrease in renal excretion [15].

PHARMACODYNAMICS

Pharmacodynamics can be defined as the study of the time course and intensity of pharmacological effects of drugs [14]. In other words, it describes what a drug does to the body. The pharmacological effects that are produced by a dose or concentration of a medication differ widely among patients. The functional relationship between concentration at a site and the intensity of the produced response follows a mathematical sigmoid or "S" pattern [14]. A marginal effect occurs at a low dose or concentration, and as the dose or concentration increases, the intensity of effect increases until a maximum effect occurs. Eventually this effect plateaus and a further increase in dose does not produce a greater effect [14]. This formula can be practically applied to clinical psychopharmacology. Each patient has a theoretical dose-response curve, and this must be kept in mind with dosage adjustments, especially with regard to where the starting point is on the curve. At a low dose or concentration, a larger dose may be necessary to achieve a therapeutic effect. An increase in dose in the linear portion of the relationship should yield a proportional increase in effect. In the higher dose or concentration area, a practitioner would probably get diminishing returns with a further increase in medication because the enzyme-binding sites or receptors will probably be saturated [14].

Medications generally have an effect on multiple receptors. For any given medication, several theoretical concentration-effect relationships are possible [14]. This pharmacodynamic effect results in inter- and intraindividual variability. An example of the importance of recognizing this variability is a concurrent general medical illness that may narrow the range of medication doses for a patient without precipitating side effects.

TOLERANCE
Sometimes the response to a medication diminishes before the concentration declines. This effect is called *tolerance*, and the time course varies from weeks to months for psychoactive medications [14]. The mechanisms involved in the development of tolerance are listed in Table 3.11 [14].

DOSE-EFFECT RELATIONSHIP VARIABILITY
The pharmacokinetic and pharmacodynamic variability presents a real challenge when treating psychiatric disorders, including the anxiety disorders. Variability in the dose-effect relationship includes active metabolites, age, weight, and disease states (Table 3.12) [14].

Most psychotropic medications (except lithium and gabapentin) are cleared partially or completely primarily by liver metabolism [14]. Many medications produce active metabolites, and the effects can be similar to or different than the parent drug. The clinician must consider the presence of active metabolites, especially

---

TABLE 3.11. Mechanisms involved in tolerance development

- Acute depletion of a neurotransmitter or cofactor
- Blockade of transporters resulting in homeostasis in receptor sensitivity
- Receptor agonist or antagonist effects

Adapted from ref. [14].

TABLE 3.12. Pharmacokinetic and pharmacodynamic variability

- Active metabolites
- Pharmacogenetics
- Combining two or more medications
- Patient noncompliance
- Physiological differences among patients
- Age
- Weight
- Disease states (e.g., liver, kidney, cardiovascular)

Adapted from ref. [14].

TABLE 3.13. Characteristics of enantiomers

Enantiomers may:
- Bind to transport proteins with different affinities
- Bind to drug-metabolizing enzymes with different affinities
- Bind to pharmacological sites of action with different affinities
- Differ in absorption
- Differ in metabolism
- Differ in protein binding
- Differ in excretion
- Modify the effects of another enantiomer

Adapted from ref. [14].

when changing from one drug or class of drugs to another [14]. The metabolites accumulate at a steady state in relation to their elimination half-lives.

For some medications, the pharmacological effect may not occur until the drug and active metabolites have all reached their steady-state concentration. For other medications that produce their effects indirectly via second messengers or a cascade of receptor actions, achieving the full effects may require an even longer period of time [14].

Many of the newer medications are single isomers, and this is true for psychoactive drugs as well. Many psychoactive drugs are two or more stereoisomers or enantiomers that have identical physicochemical properties but different biological properties [14]. They appear on the market as racemic mixtures (50:50) of both isomers. The characteristics of enantiomers that help to classify them as distinct entities are listed in Table 3.13 [14]. Single isomer medications may offer advantages over the racemic mixture (Table 3.14) [14]. An example of a single isomer antidepressant used in the treatment of anxiety disorders is escitalopram (Lexapro).

TABLE 3.14. Advantages of single isomer medications

- Less complex pharmacological profile
- More selective pharmacological profile
- Potential for improved therapeutic index
- More simplified pharmacokinetic profile
- Potential for reduced complex drug interactions
- More definable relationship between plasma drug concentration and effect

Adapted from ref. [14].

SUMMARY

Appropriate pharmacotherapy of anxiety disorders depends on the primary care practitioner's understanding and skillfully implementing various aspects of psychopharmacology. Psychopharmacology, being both an art and a science, includes a comprehensive clinical evaluation, appropriate diagnosis, determining the symptoms that are medication responsive, and a thorough discussion of the illness and treatment plan with the patient. Being comfortable with pharmacokinetic and pharmacodynamic principles allows the practitioner to individualize medications and to use them in a rational manner. The clinician must carefully monitor the patient for desired medication effects, adverse effects, as well as drug–drug interactions. Relieving patients' symptoms and improving their function equates with improving quality of life.

References

1. Venes D, ed. Taber's Cyclopedic Medical Dictionary, 20th ed. Philadelphia: F.A. Davis, 2005.
2. Stein MB. Anxiety disorders: somatic treatment. In: Sadock BJ, Sadock VA, eds. Sadock's Comprehensive Textbook of Psychiatry, 8th ed., vol. 1. Philadelphia: Lippincott Williams and Wilkins, 2005:1780–1787.
3. Davidson JRT, Connor KC. Treatment of anxiety disorders. In: Schatzberg AF, Nemeroff CB, eds. The American Psychiatric Publishing Textbook of Psychopharmacology, 3rd ed. Arlington, VA: American Psychiatric Publishing, 2004:913–934.
4. Marangell LB, Silver JM, Goff DC, Yudofsky SC. Psychopharmacology and Electroconvulsive Therapy. In: Schatzberg AF, Nemeroff CB, eds. The American Psychiatric Publishing Textbook of Psychopharmacology, 3rd ed. Arlington, VA: American Psychiatric Publishing, 2004:1047–1149.
5. Hollifield M, Mackey AM, Davidson J. Integrating therapies for anxiety disorders. Psychiatr Ann 2006;36:5:329–338.
6. Szabo ST, Gould TD, Manji HK. Neurotransmitters, receptors, signal transduction, and second messengers in psychiatric disorders. In: Schatzberg AF, Nemeroff CB, eds. The American Psychiatric

Publishing Textbook of Psychopharmacology, 3rd ed. Arlington: American Psychiatric Publishing, 2004:3–52.

7. Melchitzky DS, Austin MC, Lewis DA. Chemical Neuroanatomy of the Primate Brain. In: Schatzberg AF, Nemeroff CB, eds. The American Psychiatric Publishing Textbook of Psychopharmacology, 3rd ed. Arlington, VA: American Psychiatric Publishing, 2004:69–87.

8. Ninan PT, Muntasser S, Buspirone and gepirone. In: Schatzberg AF, Nemeroff CB, eds. The American Psychiatric Publishing Textbook of Psychopharmacology, 3rd ed. American Psychiatric Publishing, 2004:391–393.

9. Bonne O, Drevets WC, Neumeister A, Charney DS. Neurobiology of anxiety disorders. In: Schatzberg AF, Nemeroff CB, eds. The American Psychiatric Publishing Textbook of Psychopharmacology, 3rd ed. American Psychiatric Publishing, 2004:775–785.

10. Tecott LH, Smart SL. Monoamine neurotransmitters. In: Sadock BJ, Sadock VA, eds. Sadock's Comprehensive Textbook of Psychiatry, 8th ed., vol. 1. Philadelphia: Lippincott Williams & Wilkins, 2005:49–60.

11. Nemeroff CB, Putman JS. Beta-adrenergic receptor antagonists. In: Sadock BJ, Sadock VA, eds. Sadock's Comprehensive Textbook of Psychiatry, 8th ed., vol. 2. Philadelphia: Lippincott Williams & Wilkins, 2005:2722–2727.

12. Dubovsky S. Benzodiazepine receptor agonists and antagonists. In: Sadock BJ, Sadock VA, eds. Sadock's Comprehensive Textbook of Psychiatry, 8th ed., vol 2. Philadelphia: Lippincott Williams & Wilkins, 2005:2781–2791.

13. Plata-Salaman CR, Shank RP, Smith-Swintosky VL. In: Sadock BJ, Sadock VA, eds. Sadock's Comprehensive Textbook of Psychiatry, 8th ed., vol 1. Philadelphia: Lippincott Williams & Wilkins, 2005:60–68.

14. DeVane CL. Principles of pharmacokinetics and pharmacodynamics. In: Shatzberg AF, Nemeroff CB, eds. The American Psychiatric Publishing Textbook of Psychopharmacology, 3rd ed. American Psychiatric Publishing, 2004:129–145.

15. Janicac PG, Davis LM, Preskhorn, Ayd FJ. Pharmacokinetics. In: Retford DC, ed. Principles and Practice of Psychopharmacotherapy. Baltimore: Williams & Wilkins, 1993:59–79.

16. Greenblatt DJ, von Moltke LL. Pharmacokinetics and drug interactions. In: Sadock BJ, Sadock VA, eds. Sadock's Comprehensive Textbook of Psychiatry, 8th ed., vol 2. Philadelphia: Lippincott Williams & Wilkins, 2005:2699–2706.

4
Psychopharmacotherapy

John R. Vanin

HISTORY OF ANXIOLYTICS

Early anxiolytics included alcohol, bromide preparations, paraldehyde, barbiturates, and nonbarbiturates such as glutethimide, methaqualone, and methyprylon. Many of these antianxiety medications developed over the last century were thought to have fewer side effects than previous agents but proved to be highly addicting and fatal in overdose [1].

Chlordiazepoxide (Librium), the first benzodiazepine, was introduced in the late 1950s. Other benzodiazepine derivatives followed, including diazepam (Valium), oxazepam (Serax), clorazepate (Tranxene), lorazepam (Ativan), alprazolam (Xanax), and clonazepam (Klonopin).

Benzodiazepines are effective anxiolytics, widely used, and considered by many to be first-line medications for the treatment of anxiety [1,2]. Clinicians must keep in mind, however, that chronic treatment with benzodiazepines may cause psychological and physical dependence and other side effects such as sedation and psychomotor impairment [1].

Tricyclic antidepressants (TCAs) and monoamine oxidase inhibitors (MAOIs) were found to be effective anxiolytics in the 1960s. Their side-effect profiles limited their use and researchers continued to search for novel antidepressants as well as other classes of medications to treat anxiety disorders.

The first available nonsedative, nonbenzodiazepine anxiolytic was the azapirone buspirone (BuSpar) [1,3]. Buspirone showed effectiveness in the treatment of generalized anxiety disorder and did not have side effects such as dependence, psychomotor impairment, withdrawal symptoms, or lethality in overdose. However, many consider buspirone to be a relatively weak anxiolytic [1].

The selective serotonin reuptake inhibitors (SSRIs) and the serotonin-norepinephrine reuptake inhibitors (SNRIs) have been shown in controlled studies to be effective medications and many have the U.S. Food and Drug Administration (FDA) approval for the treatment of anxiety disorders [1,4]. Despite having relatively benign side effect profiles compared to TCAs and MAOIs, the SSRIs and SNRIs have a delayed onset of action, have a substantial nonresponse rate, may cause sexual dysfunction, and exhibit discontinuation syndromes with abrupt stopping [1,5,6].

Primary care practitioners may find other medications helpful, used alone or as adjunctive therapies, for certain patients with anxiety disorders, especially those who are refractory to other therapies. These medications include other antidepressants, β-adrenergic receptor antagonists, antihistamines, anticonvulsants, antipsychotics, and α_1-adrenergic antagonists [2,7,8]. Medications approved for nonpsychiatric disorders are commonly used to treat psychiatric conditions including anxiety disorders. The Food, Drug, and Cosmetic Act does not limit the way an approved medication may be used by the clinician [9]. A commercially approved medication may be prescribed "off-label" for an unapproved indication, or at a different dosage from what is listed in the package labeling [9]. When a clinician uses a medication off-label, good clinical judgment must be utilized to serve the psychiatric needs and the overall welfare of the patient.

Medications without an FDA indication are used routinely for psychiatric disorders. It is good clinical practice to explain to the patient the reason for the off-label medication use (e.g., safety, tolerability, difficult case); discuss side effects, risks, and benefits; obtain informed consent; and document the information in the patient's chart. The practitioner should be familiar with the standards of practice and the evidence-based literature supporting the effectiveness of the off-label medication [9]. Consultation with a psychiatric colleague may be helpful.

Some antidepressants are effective anxiolytics, while others have antidepressant effects without being anxiolytic. For example, bupropion (Wellbutrin) is effective for major depression with anxiety features, but it is not indicated for anxiety disorders such as panic or generalized anxiety disorder [1]. This fact is important because it stresses the importance of appropriate diagnosis as well as supports the distinctiveness of anxiety disorders as independent of mood disorders [1].

The knowledge of which medications work for anxiety disorders is often greater than the understanding of the mechanism of how they work [2]. For example, benzodiazepines are very effective anxiolytics, but when they were first developed the mechanism of action (effects on the γ-aminobutyric acid [GABA]-benzodiazepine receptor complex) was not known.

Researchers and clinicians know that many antidepressants are effective for the treatment of anxiety disorders. The mechanism of action is presumed to be similar to that of treating depression, which includes alterations in serotonin metabolism, changes in receptor sensitivity, and possibly actions of other neurotransmitters or neurotrophic factors [2]. It is important for the clinician to help the patient understand that medications do not cure anxiety disorders but can help keep the symptoms under control and allow them to have a good quality of life. This is very similar to the treatment of many common general medical disorders.

TREATMENT

A general medical and psychiatric evaluation by the primary care practitioner is the first step in the management of patients with anxiety disorders. This includes taking a careful history, performing a physical examination, and obtaining indicated laboratory and other studies. It is important to rule out medically treatable conditions, including anxiety symptoms due to medications (prescribed and nonprescribed) and other substances, as well as anxiety due to substance abuse and withdrawal.

The clinician and patient have several options in the management of anxiety disorders. Some patients prefer to cope with the anxiety symptoms, learn more via education, or utilize psychotherapy. Others prefer taking medications to correct a chemical dysregulation. Still others prefer a combination approach including pharmacotherapy, psychotherapy, and education. If the expected results of treatment are not attained in a reasonable time with a given treatment modality (e.g., sufficient dose of medication, adequate number of psychotherapy sessions, adequate length of treatment), the clinician should consider changing to an alternate form or dose of the same treatment, augment/combine, or switch to another form of treatment [2].

Anxiety disorders are usually chronic, lifelong conditions that generally do not spontaneously remit. Long-term medication treatment is often necessary and the primary care practitioner must use good clinical judgment regarding the length of treatment. There are good data showing that continued medication treatment can protect patients from relapse [10]. A practical goal for the clinician and the patient is to strive for remission of the anxiety disorder, which essentially means minimal anxiety symptoms and full function. Adequately treated patients with anxiety disorders are indistinguishable from persons without anxiety disorders [10].

PHARMACOTHERAPY

Pharmacotherapy of anxiety disorders is based on several factors. Table 4.1 lists several determining factors that a practitioner may find helpful for the pharmacotherapy of anxiety disorders [2,11].

Antidepressants

Selective Serotonin Reuptake Inhibitors

Antidepressants are among the most effective antianxiety medications. Selective serotonin reuptake inhibitors have proven efficacy for the treatment of the major anxiety disorder categories [12] and are often recommended as first-line medications. As a group, they have been shown to reduce or prevent various forms of anxiety [2]. The SSRIs have been FDA approved for indications of the different categories of anxiety disorders. The primary care clinician is increasingly taking on the duties of managing patients with anxiety disorders. Practitioners often have experience using the SSRIs as antidepressants, and so using these medications to treat anxiety disorders is very similar, including the dosages. All SSRIs are more or less effective for the common anxiety disorders [2] and have been FDA approved for specific anxiety disorder indications (Table 4.2) [12–20]. Table 4.3 lists common starting dosages, usual daily dosages, and half-lives of SSRIs [2,13–17,21].

The SSRIs inhibit the serotonin reuptake pump and increases synaptic serotonin levels. This leads to presynaptic autoreceptor downregulation, which causes an increase in the transmission of serotonin. Ultimately, there are secondary effects on signal transduction (second messenger systems) and gene transcription [21].

It is important to start treatment of anxiety disorders with lower initial dosages of SSRIs and increase slowly to a therapeutic dose.

TABLE 4.1. Factors determining anxiety disorders pharmacotherapy

- Prior patient/family response to a particular medication
- Evidence base for particular medications for particular anxiety disorders
- Side-effect profile of medication
- Practitioner comfort and experience treating anxiety disorders
- Patient preference
- Treatment algorithms/guidelines
- Cost
- Formulary restrictions

Adapted from refs. [2] and [11].

TABLE 4.2. Selective serotonin reuptake inhibitor (SSRI) treatment of anxiety disorders: U.S. Food and Drug Administration (FDA) indications

Generic (trade)	GAD	SAD	Panic	OCD	PTSD
Fluoxetine (Prozac)			+	+	
Fluvoxamine (Luvox)				+	
Sertraline (Zoloft)		+	+	+	+
Paroxetine (Paxil)	+	+	+	+	+
Paroxetine (Paxil CR)		+	+		
Citalopram (Celexa)					
Escitalopram (Lexapro)	+				

GAD, generalized anxiety disorder; OCD, obsessive-compulsive disorder; PTSD, posttraumatic stress disorder; SAD, social anxiety disorder. Adapted from refs. [12] to [20].

TABLE 4.3. SSRIs used for anxiety disorders

Generic (trade)	Starting dose (mg)	Usual daily dose (mg)	Half-life (hours) [active metabolite]
Fluoxetine (Prozac)	5–10	20–80	72 [144]
Fluvoxamine (Luvox)	50	50–300	15
Paroxetine (Paxil)	10	20–60	20
Paroxetine controlled release (Paxil CR)	12.5	25–75	20
Sertraline (Zoloft)	12.5–25	50–200	26 [66]
Citalopram (Celexa)	10	20–60	35
Escitalopram (Lexapro)	5	10–30	32

Adapted from refs. [2], [13] to [17], and [21].

This reduces the chance of increasing anxiety symptoms and minimizes the "jitteriness" syndrome that may occur with initial antidepressant medication, especially if the starting dose is too large. Starting low (perhaps 50% or less of starting dosages for depression) and increasing slowly is especially important in patients with generalized anxiety disorder and panic disorder. Standard starting doses should also be decreased by half in elderly patients and patients with other medical disorders such as liver disease.

It generally takes several weeks before anxiety disorder symptoms are alleviated with antidepressant therapy, and the patient must be aware of this. Educating patients about the disorder and treatment expectations is very important so that they will not become discouraged and will be more compliant with treatment.

A typical therapeutic trial of SSRIs may be as long as 8 to 12 weeks. The clinician should adjust the dose of medication to a therapeutic level while monitoring for desired effects and side effects. It is not unusual for patients with anxiety disorders to require doses of antidepressant medications in the higher recommended ranges. The goal, as with depression and other general medical disorders, is complete remission, not simply improvement of symptoms. Patients who are partially treated are at a greater risk for recurrence of anxiety symptoms as well as persistent functional problems [2].

If a patient does not tolerate the first SSRI because of adverse effects or if the medication is ineffective at a therapeutic dose, the clinician can switch to another SSRI, switch to another class of antidepressants, or augment or combine with another medication such as a benzodiazepine or buspirone (BuSpar) [2].

The SSRIs can be given once a day and are generally well tolerated. They lack many of the troublesome side effects associated with the older TCAs and were developed for this reason. The selectivity characteristics of SSRIs have several advantages over the TCAs including a reduction in dangerous side effects (Table 4.4) [21]. The SSRIs are unlikely to affect the seizure threshold or cardiac conduction and are much safer in overdose than TCAs [21].

The cytochrome P-450 (CYP) isoenzyme system is involved in metabolizing the SSRIs, and SSRIs may have an effect on various CYP isoenzymes as well. Table 4.5 lists examples of SSRIs and their relationships with major CYP isoenzymes [13–17,22–25]. The SSRIs are most often metabolized by CYP2C19, CYP2D6, and CYP3A4 isoenzymes [22]. Fluvoxamine (Luvox), an inhibitor of the most CYP isoenzymes of all the SSRIs, interacts with many medications [22].

The elimination of drugs and other substances can occur by multiple pathways including overlapping enzyme systems and

TABLE 4.4. Pharmacologic selectivity properties of SSRIs and tricyclic antidepressants

Action	SSRI	TCA
Muscarinic receptor blockade	–	+
H-1 histaminergic receptor blockade	–	+
α_1-adrenergic receptor blockade	–	+
Norepinephrine reuptake blockade	–	+ (especially secondary amine)
Serotonin reuptake blockade	+	+ (especially tertiary amine)

+, demonstrated property; –, largely lacking pharmacologic property.
Adapted from ref. [21].

TABLE 4.5. SSRIs and the cytochrome P-450 (CYP) enzyme system

Generic (trade)	CYP1A2	CYP2C9	CYP2C19	CYP2D6	CYP3A4
Citalopram (Celexa)	wk inh		wk inh, s	wk inh, s	s
Escitalopram (Lexapro)			s	wk inh	s
Fluoxetine (Prozac)	wk inh	s,wk/mo inh	s, mo inh	s, st inh	s, wk inh*
Fluvoxamine (Luvox)	s, st inh	wk/mo inh	mo/st inh	s, wk inh	mo inh
Paroxetine (Paxil, Paxil CR)	wk inh	wk inh	wk/mod inh	s, st inh	wk inh
Sertraline (Zoloft)**	wk inh	s, wk inh	s, wk/mo inh	s, wk/mo inh	s, wk inh

*Fluoxetine's active metabolite norfluoxetine is a moderate inhibitor.
**CYP 2B6 may contribute to metabolism.
s, substrate; wk inh, weak inhibitor; mo inh, moderate inhibitor; st inh, strong inhibitor.
Adapted from refs. [13] to [17], and [22] to [24].

TABLE 4.6. Mechanisms of potential SSRI–drug interactions

- Cytochrome enzyme inhibition
- Cytochrome enzyme induction
- Enhancement of monoamines pharmacodynamically (e.g., SSRIs used with monoamine oxidase inhibitors (MAOIs) resulting in serotonin syndrome)

Adapted from refs. [12] and [26].

alternative elimination routes [26]. This appears to be a built-in safety factor. For example, some patients have a genetic variation and are poor CYP2D6 metabolizers [27]. Because of multiple enzyme systems that metabolize the same drug, the patient with this variation may tolerate a drug usually metabolized by the CYP2D6 pathway.

The SSRIs can interact with other medications that the primary care practitioner prescribes. Mechanisms of potential interactions are listed in Table 4.6 [12,26]. Enzyme inhibition, which may result in slower elimination of another drug, resulting in an increased plasma concentration, can occur with the first dose of the inhibitor medication, and the pharmacodynamic effects may quickly change [26]. As the inhibitor is eliminated, the inhibitory effects reverse, but the effects may continue after the elimination of the inhibitor [26]. An agent that induces the cytochrome enzymes usually must be administered for days or weeks for noticeable effects, and the clinical effects of the affected drug may be gradual [26]. There may be a slow return of the affected drug concentration when the agent that caused the induction is withdrawn and the effects may last after the drug is discontinued [26].

Table 4.7 lists examples of drugs and their potential effects on or competition for the CYP system [13,15,16,22,24–26,28–31]. It is estimated that the CYP isoenzymes are responsible for the

TABLE 4.7. Examples of drugs/other substances and their relationship with several cytochrome P-450 isoenzymes

CYP1A2

acetaminophen s	haloperidol s	phenytoin ind
amiodarone i	imipramine s *	propranolol s
amitriptyline s	insulin ind	rifampin ind
β-naphthoflavone ind	interferon i	riluzole s *
broccoli ind	methadone s	ritonavir ind
brussels sprouts ind	methoxsalen i	ropivacaine s
caffeine s, i	methylcholanthrene ind	sertraline i
char grilled (charcoaled) meats ind	mexiletine s *	tacrine s * i
cimetidine i *	mibefradil i	theophylline s *
cigarette smoke ind	moclobemide i	thiabendazole i
citalopram i	modafinil ind	thiothixene s
clomipramine s	nafcillin ind	ticlopidine i *
clozapine s *	naproxen s *	tizanidine s
cruciferous vegetables ind	naringin i (grapefruit juice)	tobacco smoke ind *
cyclobenzaprine s *	olanzapine s, ind	tricyclic antidepressants (tertiary) s
duloxetine s	omeprazole ind	verapamil s
estradiol s	ondansetron s	R-warfarin s
fluoroquinolones i *	paroxetine i	zileuton s
fluoxetine i	phenacetin s	zolmitriptan s
fluvoxamine s, i *	phenobarbital ind	
furafylline i	phenothiazines s	

CYP2C9/10

amiodarone i *	irbesartan s *	probenecid i
amitriptyline s	isoniazid i *	rifampin ind *
barbiturates ind	itroconazole i	rosiglitazone s
carbamazepine ind	ketoconazole i	secobarbital ind *
celecoxib s *	lornoxicam s	sertraline inh

Continued

TABLE 4.7. *Continued*

d-propoxyphene i
diclofenac s *
disulfiram i
fenofibrate i
fluconazole i *
fluoxetine s, i
fluvastatin s*, i
fluvoxamine i
glibenclamide s
glipizide s *
glimepiride s
glyburide s
ibuprofen s *
indomethacin s

losartan s *
lovastatin i
meloxicam s
metronidazole i
miconazole i
naproxen s *
nateglinide s
norpiroxicam s
omeprazole s
paroxetine inh
phenobarbital ind
phenylbutazone i
phenytoin s*, ind
piroxicam s *

sulfamethoxazole s *, i
sulfinpyrazone i
sulfaphenazole i
suprofen s
tamoxifen s *
teniposide i
tolbutamide s *
torsemide s *
trimethoprim i
voriconazole i
S-warfarin s *
zafirlukast i

CYP2C19

amitriptyline s*
carbamazepine ind
carisoprodol s
chloramphenicol i
cimetidine i
citalopram s, i
clomipramine s *
cyclophosphamide s *
diazepam s *
escitalopram s
felbamate i
fluconazole i
fluoxetine s, i *
fluvoxamine i *
hexobarbital s
imipramine s, i

indomethacin s
ketoconazole i *
lansoprazole s *, i *
S-mephenytoin s
R-mephobarbital s
modafinil i
moclobemide s, i
nelfinavir s
nilutamide s
norethindrone ind
norphenytoin (o) s
omeprazole s *, i *
oxcarbazepine i
pantoprazole s *
paroxetine i
phenobarbitone s *

phenytoin s*, i
prednisone ind
primidone s
probenecid i
progesterone s *
proguanil s
propranolol s
rabeprazole s *
rifampin ind
rosuvastatin s
sertraline s, i
teniposide s
ticlopidine i *
topiramate i
tranylcypromine i
warfarin s

CYP2D6

alprenolol s
amiodarone i *
amitriptyline s *
amphetamine s
aripiprazole s *
atomoxetine s
beta-blockers s

bufuralol s
bupropion i *
carvedilol s
celecoxib i
chlorpheniramine s, i *
chlorpromazine s, i

duloxetine s *, i *
encainide s
escitalopram i
flecainide s *
fluoxetine s, i
fluphenazine s, i
fluvoxamine s, i
  (weak)
haloperidol s *, i *
halofantrine i
hydroxy bupropion i
hydroxyzine i
imipramine s *
levomepromazine i

perhexiline s
perphenazine s, i
phenacetin s
phenformin s
promethazine s
propafenone s *,i
propofol s

propranolol s
quinidine i *
ranitidine i
rifampin ind
risperidone s *
ritonavir i *

Continued

TABLE 4.7. *Continued*

cimetidine i *	lidocaine s	sertraline s, i (weak)
citalopram s, i	methadone i *	sparteine s
clemastine i	methoxyamphe- tamine s	tamoxifen s*
clomipramine s *, i *	metoclopramide s, i	terbinafine i
clozapine s	S-metoprolol s *	thioridazine s *, i
cocaine i	mexiletine s *	ticlopidine i
codeine */hydrocodone s	mianserin s	timolol s *
debrisoquine s	mibefradil i *	tramadol s *
d-fenfluramine s	midodrine i	trazodone s
desipramine s *	minaprine s	TCAs s
dexamethasone ind	mirtazapine s	tripelennamine i
dexfenfluramine s	moclobemide i	venlafaxine s *, i
dextromethorphan s *	nebivolol s	zuclopenthixol s
diphenhydramine i	nortriptyline s	
donepezil s	ondansetron s *	
doxepin i	oxycodone s	
doxorubicin i	paroxetine s *, i *	

CYP3A4,5,7

acetaminophen s	escitalopram s	phenobarbital ind *
alfentanil s	estrogens s	phenytoin ind *
alprazolam s *	erythromycin s *, i *	pimozide s *
amiodarone s, i *	ethosuximide s	pioglitazone ind
amitriptyline s	etoposide s	progesterone s
amlodipine s *	felodipine s *	propafenone s
amprenavir s	fentanyl s	propanolol s
androgens s	finasteride s	protease inhibitors s, i
aprepitant s, i	fluconazole i	quetiapine s
aripiprazole s *	fluoxetine i	quinidine s *
astemizole s *	fluvoxamine i *	quinine s *
atorvastatin s *	gestodene i	rifabutin ind *
barbiturates ind	Gleevec s *	rifampin ind *
buspirone s *	grapefruit juice (naringin) i *	risperidone s
cafergot s	haloperidol s * (in part)	ritonavir s *, i * ind
caffeine s	ifosfamide s	salmeterol s
calcium channel blockers s	imatinib i	saquinavir s *, i
carbamazepine s, ind *	imipramine s	sertraline s, i (weak)
cerivastatin s *	indinavir s *, i *	sildenafil s *
chloramphenicol i	irinotecan s	simvastatin s *
chlorpheniramine s *	itraconazole i *	sirolimus s
cilostazol s	ketoconazole i *	star fruit i
cimetidine i *	lercanidipine s	St. John's Wort ind *
ciprofloxacin i	lidocaine s	sufentanil s

Continued

TABLE 4.7. *Continued*

cisapride s *	loratadine s	tacrolimus s *
citalopram s	lovastatin s *	tamoxifen s *
clarithromycin s *, i *	methadone s *	Taxol s
clomipramine s	mibefradil i *	telithromycin s *, i
clonazepam s	midazolam s *	testosterone s
clozapine s	mifepristone i	terfenadine s
cocaine s	mirtazapine s	tiagabine s
codeine s	modafinil ind	topiramate ind
corticosteroids s, ind	nateglinide s	trazodone s *
cyclophosphamide s	nefazodone s, i *	triazolam s *
cyclosporine s *	nelfinavir i *	TCAs (tertiary) s
dapsone s	neviparine ind	troglitazone ind *
delavirdine i	nifedipine s *	troleandomycin i *
dexamethasone s, i, ind	nimodipine s	venlafaxine s
dextromethorphan s	nisoldipine s *	verapamil s *, i *
diazepam s *	nitrendipine s *	vinblastine s
diltiazem s, i *	norfloxacin i	vincristine s *
disopyramide s	norfluoxetine i	voriconazole i
docetaxel s	ondansetron s	zaleplon s
domperidone s	omeprazole s	ziprasidone s
donepezil s	oxcarbazepine s	zolpidem s
efavirenz ind	paclitaxel s	
eplerenone s	paroxetine i	

	CYP2B6	
bupropion s *	L-rifampin ind	phenobarbital ind
cyclophosphamide s *	S-mephenytoin s	propofol s
efavirenz s *	S-mephobarbital s	ritonavir i
fluoxetine i	methadone s *	sertraline i
fluvoxamine i	norfluoxetine i	thiotepa i
ifosfamide s *	paroxetine i	ticlopidine i

*Clinically relevant.
s, substrate; i, inhibitor; ind, inducer.
Degree of inhibition is dose-dependent for many inhibitors.
Adapted from refs. [13], [15], [16], [22], [24] to [26], and [28] to [31].

biotransformation of approximately 60% of commonly prescribed medications [28]. The drugs listed have been identified as substrates, inhibitors, or inducers of specific CYP isoenzymes. The practitioner must be aware that a particular isoenzyme may not be the main metabolic pathway, and alterations in the rate of the metabolic process caused by the isoenzyme may not necessarily have a large effect on a drug's pharmacokinetics [31]. However, a prudent clinician must consider all the medications and substances the patient is taking, keep potential interactions in mind, monitor the patient closely, and consult appropriate references and advisories as necessary.

Interactions may occur with common antidepressants because of their involvement with the CYP isoenzymes. There are limited data on antidepressant adverse drug effects related to the CYP genotype, and these are based on small studies and case reports [27]. Table 4.8 lists examples of the inhibition of CYP isoenzyme system by SSRIs and other newer antidepressants [13–17,20,24,29]. Table 4.9 lists examples of drugs that may interact with commonly used antidepressants because of their interaction with CYP isoenzymes [22,25]. Practitioners must take into account potentially dangerous drug–drug interactions by being familiar with CYP isoenzymes involved in the metabolism of various coadministered medications.

Other factors to consider regarding drug–drug interactions include the effects of food, antacids, and other substances, as well as drug protein-binding effects. The effects of food and antacids appear to be clinically insignificant for the newer antidepressants. One must remember that pharmacodynamic effects rely on the free concentration of the drug not the free plasma fraction, and so the significance of interactions from plasma protein binding interactions may be overemphasized [26].

Drug–drug interactions are based on pharmacologic principles and clinical experience, and much of the information is patient-specific. Pharmacokinetic and pharmacodynamic interactions may occur in any given patient, but the clinical consequences of the

TABLE 4.8. Inhibition of CYP Enzymes by SSRIs and other newer antidepressants

Drug	CYP 1A2	CYP 2C9	CYP2C19	CYP2D6	CYP3A4
Fluoxetine	+	++	+ to ++	+++	+
Fluvoxamine	+++	++	++/+++	+	++
Paroxetine	+	+	+ to ++	+++	+
Sertraline *	+	+	+ to ++	+/++	+
Citalopram	+	0	0	0	0
Escitalopram	0	0	0	0	0
Venlafaxine	0	0	0	0 to +	0
Mirtazapine	0	0	0	+	+
Bupropion	?	?	?	+	?

*Sertraline is a modest CYP 3A4 inducer.
0, minimal or no inhibition; + mild; ++ moderate; +++ strong.
Adapted from refs. [13] to [17], [20], [24], and [29].

TABLE 4.9. Examples of drugs that interact with Cytochrome P-450 enzymes and may interact with commonly used antidepressants

CYP 1A2

acetaminophen	haloperidol	tacrine
caffeine	olanzapine	TCAs (tertiary)
cimetidine	omeprazole	theophylline
clozapine	phenacetin	thiothixene
estradiol	phenothiazines	tobacco smoke
fluoroquinolones	R-warfarin (minor)	

CYP 2C9/10

celecoxib	lovastatin	rosiglitazone
diclofenac	naproxen	S-warfarin
fluconazole	omeprazole	tamoxifen
fluvastatin	phenobarbital	tolbutamide
ibuprofen	phenytoin	trimethoprim
isoniazid	piroxicam	
losartan	rifampin	

CYP 2C19

barbiturates	lansoprazole	progesterone
carbamazepine	omeprazole	propranolol
cimetidine	mephenytoin	rifampin
citalopram	moclobemide	TCAs (tertiary)
diazepam	norethindrone	
indomethacin	pantoprazole	

CYP 2D6

amphetamines	dextromethorphan	quinidine
alprenolol	encainide	rifampin
carvedilol	flecainide	risperidone
chlorpheniramine	haloperidol	TCAs (secondary)
cimetidine	metoprolol	timolol
codeine/hydrocodone	phenothiazines	ticlopidine
dexamethasone	propranolol	tramadol

CYP 3A4

alprazolam	cyclosporine	phenytoin
androgens	dapsone	quinidine
atorvastatin	diazepam	rifampin
azithromycin	diltiazem	simvastatin
barbiturates	estrogens	tamoxifen
calcium channel blocker	grapefruit juice	triazolam
carbamazepine	HMG CoA reductase inhib.	verapamil
cimetidine	itraconazole	zolpidem
ciprofloxacin	ketoconazole	
cisapride	macrolide antibiotics	
clonazepam	nonsedating antihistamines (not loratadine)	
corticosteroids	paclitaxel	

HMG-CoA, hepatic hydroxymethylglutaryl coenzyme A.
Adapted from refs. [22] and [25].

drug interaction are important for the primary care practitioner to recognize and evaluate. The clinician must always keep potential drug–drug interactions in mind when using the SSRIs, but while serious interactions are indeed possible, dangerous and life-threatening medication interactions appear to be rare [26]. Essential drug interactions with SSRIs that a clinician must be aware of include MAOIs, TCAs, other SSRIs/antidepressants, tryptophan, dextromethorphan, theophylline, triptans, and warfarin [25,26].

When combining medications, it is important for the clinician to carefully monitor the patient for effects and side effects. Table 4.10 lists highlights for prescribing antidepressants and potential drug interactions [26].

The SSRIs are structurally different, and patients may or may not respond to one SSRI versus another. Despite their differences, the SSRIs are similar in their broad-spectrum efficacy and side-effect profiles [2,21]. They are very helpful when treating patients with anxiety disorders as well as comorbid conditions such as

TABLE 4.10. Prescribing highlights regarding potential antidepressant-drug interactions

- Be aware of well-documented interactions that are potentially clinically significant
- Learn how the major drugs prescribed are eliminated (main pathways)
- Assign risk to potential adverse drug interactions that are likely to affect therapeutic outcome and rank important variables (e.g., age, general health status, comorbid conditions)
- Determine a patient's past experiences with certain medications/substances (past problems often predict future problems)
- Vary peak concentrations by prescribing medications at different times
- Determine risk of drug–drug interactions vs. risk of not treating
- Follow target symptoms during treatment (outcome measures)
- Consider drug–drug interactions as possible reason for an inadequate response
- Try not to change more than one drug variable at a time when trying to determine specific drug side effects or changes in symptoms
- Note the expected half-life of prescribed medications when changing drug variables (e.g., drug accumulation or washout times)
- Add drugs in a stepwise manner to a current regimen
- When stopping a drug, taper if possible prior to discontinuing
- Use multiple drugs only if warranted (rational polypharmacy)
- Patient education is extremely important
- Maintain close contact with patient, especially early in treatment

Adapted from ref. [26].

depression. Many SSRI side effects are more prominent with initial treatment such as gastrointestinal effects, headaches, and insomnia, and these tend to improve with continued treatment (Table 4.11) [2,21]. Sexual dysfunction, which is common with long-term SSRI use and may not diminish over time, can be a real problem and can affect medication compliance. Sexual side effects include decreased libido, anorgasmia, erectile dysfunction, and delayed ejaculation. It is important for the clinician to assess the patient's sexual concerns prior to prescribing any of the SSRIs. Management strategies for sexual side effects are listed in Table 4.12 [21,32,33].

TABLE 4.11. SSRI side effects

nausea +	anxiety +	light-headedness
loose bowel movements/ diarrhea +	sweating +	vivid dreams
headaches +	weight loss/gain	rash
insomnia +	sexual dysfunction	discontinuation syndrome
sedation +	muscle tension	apathy syndrome
tremor	akathisia	dystonia
exacerbation of Parkinson's disease	serotonin syndrome*	drug interactions
syndrome of inappropriate secretion of antidiuretic hormone (SIADH)-esp. elderly		

*Serotonin syndrome includes mental status changes, gastrointestinal symptoms, autonomic instability, neuromuscular symptoms.
+, frequent initial side effects, usually dosage related, generally improve after first few weeks of treatment.
Adapted from refs. [2] and [21].

TABLE 4.12. Management strategies for SSRI sexual side effects

- Dose adjustments: gradual reduction of dosage may be helpful; caution any signs of relapse or discontinuation symptoms
- Drug holidays: most easily accomplished with shorter half-life medications but can lead to treatment noncompliance; caution discontinuation symptoms or relapse of symptoms
- Drug substitution: caution because equivalent therapeutic response may not occur
- Antidotal therapy to counteract SSRI side effect (e.g., buspirone, bupropion, sildenafil)
- Nonpharmacologic treatment such as psychotherapy, sex therapy

Adapted from refs. [21] and [33].

Discontinuation of Selective Serotonin Reuptake Inhibitors

Abrupt termination of SSRIs may result in a discontinuation syndrome (Table 4.13) [6]. Discontinuation syndromes have been reported with other antidepressant classes including SNRIs, TCAs, and MAOIs [6]. Medications with a relatively long half-life, such as fluoxetine offer greater protection from discontinuation syndrome [13]. It is important for the patient to know that missed doses may precipitate discontinuation symptoms [6]. A supervised discontinuation strategy is prudent with gradual tapering of the medication dosage. With gradual tapering of the medication, the patient must be aware that discontinuation symptoms are still possible and may actually be prolonged [6], although, it is hoped, less severe. Discontinuation symptoms generally last less than 3 weeks [6]. One method of management beyond a "wait and watch" approach is to increase the dose of medication again and then taper much more slowly. Also, a switch to a longer-acting medication with a gradual tapering of the dosage may be helpful.

Pregnancy and Lactation

The primary care practitioner must consider the welfare of both the mother and the child when managing psychiatric disorders such as anxiety disorders in pregnancy and lactation. This is a complex clinical situation that may involve consultants, such as the patient's obstetrician. The literature regarding the reproductive safety of psychotropic medications continues to grow, but there are few definitive data regarding authoritative guidelines for treatment during pregnancy and lactation [34]. Clinicians must carefully conduct a risk-benefit assessment regarding the anxiety disorder and treatment alternatives.

Pathways of offspring exposure include direct exposure (direct contact of any biological or pharmacological agent) and indirect exposure (an agent's influence on the environment) [34]. The potential benefits and risk of treatment with antidepressants in

TABLE 4.13. Examples of discontinuation symptoms

vertigo	shock-like reaction	ataxia	flushing
dizziness	nausea	visual changes	insomnia
light-headedness	vomiting	anxiety	fatigue
faintness	diarrhea	irritability	chills
headache	anorexia	depressed mood	vivid dreams
paresthesias	tremor	sweating	
myalgias	myoclonus	suicidal ideation intensification	

Adapted from ref. [6].

pregnancy should be carefully considered, discussed with the patient, and documented. A comprehensive discussion includes a consideration of nonpharmacological treatment, antidepressant treatment, as well as treatment discontinuation.

Based on older studies (1990s), it appeared that SSRIs were relatively safe during gestation. Newport et al. [34] summarized published reports of SSRI use during gestation and concluded there was no evidence from the data of an increased incidence of congenital malformations associated with prenatal exposure. Pies discussed a study by Pastuszak et al. in the 1990s which found no evidence of teratogenicity compared with matched controls in 128 women taking fluoxetine during the first trimester [35]. These data are reassuring, but safety data for several newer antidepressants is limited [36]. Exposure to antidepressants in utero also resulted in little long-term neurobehavioral risk to children according to several studies, but these results appear to be inconclusive and speculative because of study limitations [35,36]. According to data from the last several years, the general overall safety of SSRIs and related antidepressants during pregnancy is still supported but there have been some concerns [35].

The FDA has issued a public health advisory about exposure to paroxetine during the first trimester and the risk of cardiac congenital malformations. Paroxetine's pregnancy category was reclassified from a C to a D [35–37] (Table 4.14) [20,23,34,35]. Numerous limitations in the data set make it difficult to draw definitive conclusions about this analysis [36]. Pies, Zing et al., and

TABLE 4.14. U.S. FDA pregnancy categories and nursing cautions of SSRIs and other antidepressants

Generic (trade)	Pregnancy category*	Nursing information
Fluoxetine (Prozac)	C	Not for use in nursing
Sertraline (Zoloft)	C	Caution in nursing
Paroxetine (Paxil, Paxil CR)	D	Caution in nursing
Citalopram (Celexa)	C	Not for use in nursing
Escitalopram (Lexapro)	C	Not for use in nursing
Venlafaxine extended release (Effexor XR)	C	Not for use in nursing

*Pregnancy category C: risk cannot be ruled out; human studies are lacking, and animal studies are either positive for fetal risk or lacking as well; potential benefits may justify the potential risk.
*Pregnancy category D: positive evidence of risk; investigational or post-marketing data show risk to fetus; potential benefits may outweigh risks.
Adapted from refs. [20], [23], [34], and [35].

an FDA Health Advisory cited a retrospective case control study, which reported a significant association between the use of SSRIs after the 20th week of pregnancy and the presence of persistent pulmonary hypertension of the newborn [35–37]. Despite statistical significance, questions have been raised regarding the clinical meaningfulness [36]. There have also been increased reports of neonatal abstinence syndrome associated with SSRIs; however, this syndrome is generally mild and self-limiting [35].

Clinically, the primary care practitioner must carefully evaluate each patient and weigh the effects and risk of untreated maternal anxiety disorders against the risk of fetal exposure to antidepressant medications [36]. There is some evidence that anxiety disorders can affect pregnancy outcomes [38]. Comorbid psychiatric conditions such as depression often occur with anxiety disorders as well.

A conservative approach regarding medications is always prudent. If possible, nonpharmacological treatment (e.g., cognitive-behavioral therapy, psychosocial support, avoidance of substances such as caffeine and alcohol) should be the first-line treatment in pregnant women with anxiety disorders, including generalized anxiety disorder (GAD) and panic disorder (Table 4.15) [38]. If antidepressant therapy is warranted, it is important to choose a medication that has shown efficacy for anxiety disorders and has an extensive reproductive safety database, and to prescribe doses as low as possible to maintain clinical efficacy [36].

The American Psychiatric Association Committee on Research on Psychiatric Treatments issued a position paper on risk-benefit

TABLE 4.15. General guidelines for treatment of panic disorder and generalized anxiety disorder in pregnancy

- Use nonpharmacologic treatment whenever possible (e.g., CBT)
- SSRIs are first-line medication treatment for anxiety disorders; if medication is required, prescribe lowest effective dose for minimum amount of time
- Options for patients unresponsive or intolerant to SSRIs include newer antidepressants such as venlafaxine extended release and mirtazapine
- Avoid benzodiazepines if alternative treatments are available (e.g., SSRIs)
- Tapering medications with adjunctive CBT may be attempted if necessary to minimize fetal exposure; abrupt discontinuation of antipanic medication is not recommended
- Because the postpartum period is a high risk relapse period, women should consider postpartum resumption if medications were avoided during pregnancy

CBT, cognitive behavior therapy.
Adapted from ref. [38].

decision making for major depression during pregnancy [39]. The conclusions were that there was no evidence to implicate antidepressants as causing harm to an unborn baby, and that as long as the benefits and possible risks are explained well, a pregnant woman should be treated. Although this statement pertains specifically to the treatment of depression in pregnancy, it can perhaps be helpful for the primary care practitioner in the clinical decision making for anxiety disorders.

At this time, the FDA recommends counseling child-bearing age women about the heightened risks of birth defects associated with paroxetine during pregnancy and switching them to another antidepressant if possible [40]. The American College of Obstetricians and Gynecologists Committee on Obstetrics Practice recommends pregnant women and women planning pregnancy avoid paroxetine if possible because it may cause fetal cardiac malformations [41]. The committee also recommends an individualized approach to treating pregnant women or women who are planning pregnancy, with all SSRIs and SNRIs [41].

Studies have shown that citalopram and fluoxetine are excreted in breast milk in levels that may significantly expose a nursing infant to the SSRI. Paroxetine, fluvoxamine, and sertraline are excreted in breast milk only to a minor extent [42]. Despite overall evidence that infant exposure to SSRIs in breast milk suggests minimal risk, if treating a nursing mother is warranted, using the lowest effective dose of an SSRI that is minimally excreted in breast milk would be prudent [42].

Serotonin-Norepinephrine Reuptake Inhibitors

Serotonin-norepinephrine reuptake inhibitors are dual reuptake inhibitors. Along with SSRIs, SNRIs are considered first-line agents for the treatment of anxiety disorders. The SNRIs are efficacious for the anxiety disorders as well as depressive symptoms and have a better tolerability than the TCAs or the MAOIs [2,43]. They can be used as initial treatment or as a class of medications for the practitioner to switch to. The two SNRIs currently marketed in the U.S. are venlafaxine extended release (Effexor XR) and duloxetine (Cymbalta). Antidepressants such as imipramine and clomipramine could be considered SNRIs but are not selective and they have a potential for more side effects because of a higher affinity for other neurotransmitter receptors (Table 4.16) [44,45].

Venlafaxine XR was the first SNRI approved by the FDA for the treatment of anxiety disorders (Table 4.17) [23], and was the first FDA-approved medication for the long-term treatment of generalized anxiety disorder [4].

TABLE 4.16. Serotonin norepinephrine reuptake inhibitors (SNRIs)

Amitriptyline	Clomipramine
Imipramine	Venlafaxine
Doxepin	Duloxetine
Trimipramine	Milnacipran (not available in U.S.)

Adapted from refs. [44] and [45].

TABLE 4.17. Venlafaxine XR: U. S. FDA anxiety disorders indications

- Generalized anxiety disorder
- Social anxiety disorder (generalized)
- Panic disorder

Adapted from refs. [23].

TABLE 4.18. Venlafaxine and the CYP enzyme system

CYP1A2	CYP2C9	CYP2C19	CYP2D6	CYP3A4
–	–	–	s, wk inh	s

s, substrate; wk inh, weak inhibitor.
Adapted from refs. [22], [23], and [44].

TABLE 4.19. Examples of venlafaxine–drug interactions

- Cimetidine: may cause increase in venlafaxine levels (minimal)
- Haloperidol: may cause increase haloperidol levels
- SSRIs: may increase venlafaxine levels with risk of serotonin syndrome
- MAOIs: risk of serotonin syndrome-contraindicated
- Indinavir (Crixivan): may decrease the protease inhibitor concentration

Adapted from refs. [25], [26], and [44].

Duloxetine (Cymbalta), another SNRI currently marketed in the U.S., has clinical benefits for anxiety [46] and was recently FDA approved for the treatment of generalized anxiety disorder. Depression studies have shown significant anxiety score decreases with its use [19].

Venlafaxine is rapidly and well absorbed. The extent of absorption is not affected by food, but the rate decreases. It undergoes extensive first-pass metabolism by the CYP enzyme system, particularly CYP2D6. It is a weak CYP2D6 inhibitor as well (Table 4.18) [22,23,44]. Venlafaxine has a low potential for CYP-mediated drug–drug interactions [44]. Table 4.19 lists examples of cautions and contraindications regarding venlafaxine use with other drugs [25,26,44].

Over a dosage range of 75 to 450 mg/day, venlafaxine and its metabolite exhibit linear kinetics [44]. At therapeutic concentrations (steady state reached in 3 to 4 days), both venlafaxine and its metabolite are minimally protein bound [44]. Venlafaxine may be given once a day. either in the morning or the evening. Renal excretion is the primary excretion route and clearance may be reduced in patients with severe renal disease or cirrhosis. Starting low and increasing the dose slowly is important when treating patients with anxiety disorders, medically complicated patients, and the elderly. For example, starting venlafaxine XR at 37.5 mg/day with at least 1 week between adjustments may be prudent in this population (Table 4.20) [44].

Venlafaxine inhibits the reuptake of serotonin and norepinephrine. At lower doses, it has a higher effect on serotonin reuptake than norepinephrine reuptake [46]. Venlafaxine is probably an SSRI at low therapeutic doses and has a more balanced serotonin and norepinephrine reuptake effect at higher doses [44,46]. Venlafaxine XR has a similar side effect profile to the SSRIs (Table 4.21) [44].

Early adverse effects tend to markedly diminish with long-term treatment. Long-term adverse effects include hypertension and sexual dysfunction. Routine blood pressure monitoring is recommended, especially at the upper therapeutic range ($\geq$225 mg/day) because of potential dose-related hypertension in some patients [44]. The clinician should record blood pressure before starting the medication and monitor regularly. Venlafaxine is classified as pregnancy category C by the *Physicians' Desk Reference* (PDR) and is not for use in nursing (Table 4.14) [23].

TABLE 4.20. Venlafaxine XR use in anxiety disorders

Generic (trade)	Starting dose (mg)	Usual daily dose (mg)	Half-life (hours) [active metabolite]
Venlafaxine extended release (Effexor XR)	37.5	75–225	4 [10]

Adapted from ref. [44].

TABLE 4.21. Venlafaxine: side effects

Nausea (most common)	Headache	Hypertension
Dizziness	Dry mouth	Sexual dysfunction
Insomnia	Constipation	Nervousness
Somnolence	Sweating	Asthenia

Adapted from ref. [44].

TABLE 4.22. Venlafaxine discontinuation symptoms

Dizziness	Nausea	Diarrhea
Light-headedness	Vomiting	Nervousness
Tinnitus	Appetite loss	Sensory disturbances
Insomnia	Dry mouth	
Somnolence	Sweating	

Adapted from refs. [4] and [44].

Abrupt discontinuation of venlafaxine may be associated with several unpleasant side effects, especially at higher dosages (Table 4.22) [4,44]. The practitioner must caution the patient not to discontinue longer-term use of venlafaxine abruptly. Whenever possible, a tapering schedule of no more than 75 mg/day/week is prudent, and slower tapering may be necessary depending on the dose, the duration of therapy, and the particular patient [44].

Benzodiazepines
Benzodiazepines are among the most widely prescribed psychiatric medications [47,48]. The first benzodiazepines introduced were chlordiazepoxide (Librium) and diazepam (Valium) in 1959 and 1963, respectively. Since that time, numerous other benzodiazepines have been marketed. The triazolobenzodiazepine alprazolam (Xanax) was introduced in 1981 and it was the first benzodiazepine approved by the FDA for the treatment of panic disorder. Clonazepam (Klonopin) also is indicated for the treatment of panic disorder. Other benzodiazepines are indicated for the management of anxiety (Table 4.23) [20,47].

Considered effective and relatively safe when compared to older antianxiety medications such as barbiturates, benzodiazepines were a widely prescribed first-line treatment as anxiolytics for many years until SSRIs became available [47]. Despite their potential for dependency, withdrawal, abuse, and alcohol interaction, benzodiazepines are very useful medications in the treatment of anxiety and specific anxiety disorders, and they are pharmacologically the most effective acute antianxiety medications [47,48].

Benzodiazepines may be used in many different ways. They may be used adjunctively with antidepressants such as SSRIs and SNRIs (especially early in the course of treatment) as well as a primary treatment of anxiety symptoms that interfere with normal functioning for patients intolerant to antidepressants (Table 4.24) [2,47,49]. For example, adjunctive use of benzodiazepines with antidepressants in panic disorder may improve the therapeutic effect and help relieve the side effects such as early activation or

TABLE 4.23. U.S. FDA-approved indications for benzodiazepines

Generic (trade)	FDA indications
Alprazolam (Xanax)	Management of anxiety disorders and short-term relief of anxiety symptoms; treatment of panic disorder with/without agoraphobia
Alprazolam XR (Xanax XR)	Panic disorder with/without agoraphobia
Clonazepam (Klonopin)	Panic disorder with/without agoraphobia
Lorazepam (Ativan)	Management of anxiety
Chlordiazepoxide (Librium)	Management of anxiety disorders and short term relief of anxiety symptoms
Diazepam (Valium)	Management of anxiety disorders and short term relief of anxiety symptoms
Oxazepam (Serax)	Management of anxiety
Clorazepate (Tranxene)	Management of anxiety disorders

Adapted from refs. [20] and [47].

TABLE 4.24. Benzodiazepine use in anxiety and anxiety disorders

- Adjunctive treatment with antidepressants, especially to minimize early side effects
- As needed (prn) treatment in situational anxiety interfering with normal functioning
- Primary treatment of patients intolerant of other treatment such as antidepressants
- Primary/adjunctive treatment in patients with no/partial anxiolytic response to antidepressants

Adapted from refs. [2], [47], and [49].

jitteriness. A gradual tapering of the benzodiazepine as the antidepressant takes effect can be attempted.

Raj and Sheehan cite a 12-week study by Goddard et al. in 2001 that looked at open-label sertraline (Zoloft) and double-blind clonazepam or placebo use [47]. Adjunct medications (clonazepam or placebo) were tapered and discontinued over 3 weeks after 4 weeks of combination therapy. All patients received sertraline treatment only for the last month of the study. Results showed the sertraline/clonazepam group had fewer dropouts and separated from the sertraline-placebo group as early as week one on the Panic Disorder Severity Scale.

Benzodiazepines have a greater effect on some anxiety disorders than others. They are regularly used for the treatment of GAD, panic disorder, and generalized social anxiety disorder, but

TABLE 4.25. Expert anxiety pharmacotherapists consensus summary: potential for therapeutic benzodiazepine dose dependence and abuse

- Among the benzodiazepines, there is little consensus regarding the relative risk of dependence and abuse
- Benzodiazepines have a higher risk of dependence and abuse than most potential substitutes, but have a lower risk than older sedatives and recognized drugs of abuse
- When comparing benzodiazepine tapering vs. abrupt discontinuation, the differences between shorter and longer half-lives in causing withdrawal symptoms are less clear
- When determining the most important factors contributing to benzodiazepine withdrawal symptoms and failure to discontinue, there is little agreement
- The most important contributors to withdrawal symptoms are the medication's pharmacologic properties
- The most important contributors to medication discontinuation failure may be a patient's clinical characteristics

Adapted from ref. [48].

are not primary treatment for obsessive-compulsive disorder and posttraumatic stress disorder [2,47]. Alprazolam and clonazepam have been extensively studied in panic disorder and social anxiety disorder [2]. Concerns regarding benzodiazepine use and liability for abuse (especially with long-term use) and dependence continue, however. In 1999, a panel of experts acknowledged some abuse potential of benzodiazepines, but recommended their use for anxiety disorders even for long periods (Table 4.25) [48]. Most studies suggest that the majority of patients, over time, stay at the same dose or decrease benzodiazepine doses and maintain benefits [48]. It is important for the practitioner to note that benzodiazepines are not efficacious for major depression and may actually make depressive symptoms worse.

Clinical Characteristics
All benzodiazepines exhibit some degree of anxiolytic, sedative-hypnotic, muscle relaxant, and anticonvulsant properties. Compared to other antianxiety alternatives, benzodiazepines are clinically easier to use, have a quicker onset of action, and are generally well tolerated. These characteristics allow for better patient compliance. They can also be used on an as-needed basis (prn) for situational anxiety. Benzodiazepines are very helpful medications when acutely anxious patients need immediate treatment to provide relief from their severe, distressing, and sometimes disabling

TABLE 4.26. Benzodiazepines: dosages for anxiety and anxiety disorders

Generic (trade)	Examples
Alprazolam (Xanax)	Initial: 0.25–0.5 mg tid; may increase q3–4d; max 4 mg/d
	Initial for elderly, debilitated, advanced liver disease: 0.25 mg bid-tid. Increase gradually as tolerated
	Panic disorder: initial: 0.5 mg tid; increase by no more than 1 mg/d q3–4d; slower titration if ≥4 mg/d; usual dose: 1–10 mg/d; discontinuation: decrease slowly, no faster than 0.5 mg q3d
Alprazolam extended release (Xanax XR)	Initial: 0.5–1.0 mg (preferably q a.m.); increase by no more than 1 mg/d q3–4d; maintenance: 1–10 mg/d; usual dose: 3–6 mg/d; discontinuation: decrease dose slowly (no more than 0.5 mg q3d)
Clonazepam (Klonopin)	For panic: initial: 0.25 mg bid; after 3d increase to target dose of 1 mg/d; if necessary, increase by 0.125–0.25 mg bid q3d to a max of 4 mg/d; discontinue gradually: decrease by 0.125 mg bid q3d; wafer: dissolve in mouth with/without water
Lorazepam (Ativan)	Initial: 2–3 mg/d given bid-tid; usual dose: 2–6 mg/d, divided doses; elderly/debilitated: 1–2 mg/d divided doses
Chlordiazepoxide (Librium)	Usual daily dose for mild-mod anxiety: 5–10 mg PO tid-qid; severe anxiety: 20–25 mg PO tid-qid
Oxazepam (Serax)	Mild-mod anxiety: 10–15 mg tid-qid; severe anxiety: 15–30 mg tid-qid; elderly: initial: 10 mg tid; increase to 15 mg tid-qid
Clorazepate (Tranxene)	Initial: 15 mg h.s.; usual: 30 mg/d-divided; max dose: 60 mg/d

Adapted from refs. [20] and [23].

symptoms. Table 4.26 lists examples of benzodiazepine dosing for anxiety and anxiety disorders [20,23].

Mechanism of Action

Benzodiazepines cause antianxiety effects by their action at the GABA-benzodiazepine receptor complex. They potentiate the effects of GABA, which is the primary central nervous system inhibitory transmitter [50,51]. The clinical result is relaxation and mild sedation. GABA has two receptors: GABA-A and GABA-B. GABA-A controls the chloride-ion channel [47]. A number of receptors close to GABA-A can modulate the GABA-A receptor including benzodiazepines, nonbenzodiazepine sedatives, and alcohol [47].

When GABA occupies the GABA-A receptor site, the chloride channel opens and causes an inhibitory effect. If a benzodiazepine binds to a nearby benzodiazepine receptor, the GABA-A receptor is modulated and there is a greater effect on the chloride channel and the conductance by GABA [47]. GABA can work by itself on the GABA receptor, but benzodiazepines cannot affect the chloride channel by itself in the absence of GABA.

Pharmacokinetics

Benzodiazepines vary regarding their absorption from the gastrointestinal tract. For example, diazepam (Valium) is rapidly absorbed and acts quickly, while lorazepam (Ativan) has an intermediate absorption rate and onset of action. When given intramuscularly (IM), benzodiazepine absorption varies as well. For example, compared to chlordiazepoxide (Librium), IM lorazepam (Ativan) is more rapidly, completely, and reliably absorbed [47].

All benzodiazepine are highly lipophilic (lipid soluble) but they differ in their degree of passage across the blood–brain barrier. The quickness and intensity of onset thus varies among the different benzodiazepines. The rate and extent of drug distribution determines the duration of benzodiazepine action rather than the elimination rate (Z). The half-life of a particular benzodiazepine affects the speed and extent of accumulation, time to reach steady state, and the washout time (Table 4.27) [23,47]. Drowsiness and sedation may occur with longer half-life benzodiazepines because of greater drug accumulation [47]. Choosing a medication with a short to intermediate half-life is important for the clinician to consider in treating patients who have to remain alert, such as patients in certain jobs such as operating equipment, or those attending school, or in treating the elderly.

TABLE 4.27. Benzodiazepine pharmacokinetics

Drug	Metabolism	CYP isoenzyme	Half-life (hours)
Alprazolam	Oxidation	3A4	10–15
Clonazepam	Oxidation	?3A4	24–56
Lorazepam	Glucuronidation		10–20
Diazepam	Oxidation	2C19,3A4	26–50
Chlordiazepoxide	Oxidation	3A4	>21
Oxazepam	Glucuronidation		5–15

Adapted from refs. [23] and [47].

Benzodiazepines are metabolized by microsomal oxidation, reduction, or glucuronide conjugation in the liver. Several factors can affect the oxidative pathway including age, medical illness (e.g., liver disease), and other drugs [47]. Benzodiazepines that are conjugated (e.g., oxazepam, lorazepam) are safer than those metabolized by oxidation (e.g., alprazolam, diazepam) in elderly patients and those with medical illness such as liver disease [47].

Adverse Effects

Although benzodiazepines are among the safest psychotropic medications, side effects do occur (Table 4.28) [47,48]. Drowsiness and sedation are among the most common side effects. Long-term side effects include physiological dependence, abuse liability in predisposed individuals, and discontinuation/withdrawal symptoms. Meta-analysis of peer-reviewed studies found evidence of cognitive dysfunction in patients treated with benzodiazepines long-term [52]. Findings suggest patients should be advised of potential long-term treatment cognitive effects, but also that the impact on daily functioning of most patients may be insignificant [52]. Lack of credible controls has been a critical issue in many studies assessing long-term benzodiazepine use and cognitive effects [48].

Drug Interactions

Inhibitors of the oxidase system that metabolizes many benzodiazepines increase the half-life and may cause symptoms such as sedation, slurred speech, ataxia, and imbalance (Table 4.29) [47]. Drugs such as phenytoin and barbiturates cause liver enzyme induction, thereby reducing the half-life of benzodiazepines [47]. Benzodiazepines prolong the partial thromboplastin time (PTT) and increase digoxin levels. Antidepressants that inhibit the CYP3A4

TABLE 4.28. Benzodiazepine side effects

Drowsiness/sedation	Hostility
Ataxia	Disinhibition
Impairment of psychomotor performance	Increased dreaming
Anterograde amnesia	Sexual dysfunction
Cognitive effects	Physiologic dependence
Hyperexcitability	Abuse liability in predisposed individuals
Rebound anxiety	Discontinuation/withdrawal symptoms
Nervousness	Negative interaction with alcohol

Adapted from refs. [47] and [48].

TABLE 4.29. Examples of drugs that inhibit oxidative capacity of benzodiazepines

- Cimetidine
- Estrogens (oral contraceptives)
- MAOIs

Adapted from ref. [47].

enzyme (e.g., fluoxetine) inhibit triazolobenzodiazepine metabolism (e.g., alprazolam).

Patients with nausea and vomiting who take benzodiazepines have an increased risk for aspiration since benzodiazepines can inhibit the gag reflex [47]. Antacids containing aluminum delay gastric emptying and slow benzodiazepine absorption [47]. The clinician must also recall that in the elderly, there is decreased clearance, an increase in medication half-life, and an increase in volume of distribution [47].

Tolerance

Patients may require dosage adjustment because of the loss of some of the benefits due to tolerance [47]. A decrease in side effects may also occur due to tolerance. It may take several adjustments to reach final effective dosages, and this must not be misinterpreted as addictive behavior. Different benzodiazepines have different timelines for tolerance development with long half-life medications taking a month or longer and the shorter half-life medications exhibiting tolerance sooner, perhaps within a week [47]. Although cross-tolerance between benzodiazepines is relatively good, the clinician should not abruptly switch patients from one benzodiazepine to another [47]. Substituting a long-acting for a short-acting benzodiazepine is a common practice for detoxifying a patient addicted to a benzodiazepine (Table 4.30) [53]. Gradual reduction of dosage with discontinuation depends on several factors including dosage and duration of benzodiazepine use and severity of addiction [53].

Physical Dependence, Discontinuation, and Abuse

Long-term therapeutic benzodiazepine use can produce physical dependence [54]. Dependence implies a need for tapering the medication when discontinuing because of receptor adaptation and suppression of symptoms [48]. The clinician must recognize the difference between physical dependence and abuse. Abuse is defined as a chronic disorder, associated with compulsive drug use resulting in psychological, physical, or social harm and continued use despite

TABLE 4.30. Benzodiazepine dose equivalency (approximate)

Generic (rade)	Dose equivalents (mg.)	Short or long acting
Alprazolam (Xanax)	1	Short
Clonazepam (Klonopin)	0.5	Long
Lorazepam (Ativan)	2	Short
Chlordiazepoxide (Librium)	25	Long
Diazepam (Valium)	10	Long
Oxazepam (Serax)	30	Short

Adapted from ref. [53].

TABLE 4.31. Benzodiazepine discontinuation symptoms

Restlessness	Nausea
Irritability	Runny nose
Muscle tension	Hypersensitivity to stimuli
Tremor	Insomnia
Sweating	Agitation
*Severe withdrawal symptoms:**	
Psychosis	Paranoid delusions
Seizures	Tinnitus
Hallucinations	

*Relatively rare; more likely with abrupt withdrawal from high doses of high potency benzodiazepines and in the elderly. Adapted from refs. [47] and [54].

that harm. Part of the abuse definition includes drug seeking and difficulty in stopping drug use [47]. Physical dependence does not imply lack of benefit, abuse, or drug seeking. Benzodiazepines are not considered addictive drugs by the above criteria.

Benzodiazepine discontinuation symptoms include restlessness, irritability, muscle tension, and tremor (Table 4.31) [47,54] Factors associated with withdrawal symptoms include the dose of a drug, potency, length of use, and discontinuation rate [47]. Discontinuation syndrome occurs earlier and is more severe after abruptly stopping therapeutic doses of short-acting benzodiazepines than after stopping long-acting benzodiazepines [54]. It is prudent to slowly taper benzodiazepines (especially short-acting) when discontinuing these medications after a therapeutic course especially if used for more than 3 to 6 weeks [54]. This minimizes the development of rebound symptoms, reduces uncomfortable discontinuation symptoms, and reduces the danger of withdrawal seizures. For example, tapering alprazolam or clonazepam at a rate no faster than 0.5 mg every

2 weeks minimizes any withdrawal seizures [47]. There is generally no clinical reason to taper more quickly, and the slower withdrawal schedule may be better tolerated.

As discussed in the other sections of this chapter, many classes of medications including SSRIs, TCAs, and beta-blockers can exhibit discontinuation syndrome. The American Psychiatric Association Task Force on Benzodiazepines (1990) concluded that benzodiazepines are not drugs of abuse, although benzodiazepine abuse is common among individuals actively abusing other substances such as alcohol, opiates, sedative hypnotics, and cocaine [48]. Other evidence suggests that the abuse potential is well known and accepted, but benzodiazepine abuse is uncommon except among abusers of alcohol and other drugs [47].

Pregnancy

Teratogenic effects have been associated with benzodiazepine use in pregnancy, but these effects are controversial [47]. Problems such as oral clefts, skeletal abnormalities, pyloric stenosis, inguinal hernias, hemangiomas, and cardiovascular defects have been reported with first- and second-trimester use, but other data do not support an association between malformations and fetal exposure to benzodiazepines [47]. Tables 4.32 and 4.33 list pregnancy and nursing information regarding the benzodiazepines [20,25,47].

TABLE 4.32. Benzodiazepines: pregnancy and nursing

Generic (trade)	Pregnancy	Nursing
Alprazolam (Xanax)	Category D	Not for use in nursing
Alprazolam extended release (Xanax XR)	Category D	Not for use in nursing
Clonazepam (Klonopin)	Category D	Not for use in nursing
Clonazepam orally disintegrating tabs (Klonopin Wafers)	Category D	Not for use in nursing
Chlordiazepoxide (Librium)	Not for use in pregnancy	Safety in nursing not known
Diazepam (Valium)	Not for use in pregnancy	Safety in nursing not known
Lorazepam (Ativan)	Not for use in pregnancy	Not for use in nursing
Oxazepam (Serax)	Not for use in pregnancy	Not for use in nursing
Clorazepate (Tranxene)	Safety in pregnancy not known	Not for use in nursing

Adapted from refs. [20], [25], and [47].

TABLE 4.33. Benzodiazepines and pregnancy: general concerns

- According to suggestions by several studies, there is an increased risk of congenital malformations associated with benzodiazepine use in pregnancy
- Benzodiazepine use should almost always be avoided during pregnancy especially the first trimester
- Nonteratogenic risks in children born to mothers taking benzodiazepines during pregnancy include reports of:
  - flaccidity
  - respiratory difficulties
  - feeding difficulties
  - hypothermia
- There are reports of children born to mothers who took benzodiazepines late in pregnancy experiencing withdrawal symptoms during postnatal period

Adapted from refs. [20], [25], and [47].

Central nervous system depression and withdrawal symptoms may occur when benzodiazepines are used in the third trimester and through delivery, and neonatal withdrawal symptoms may be present at birth or may appear weeks later [47]. Neonatal symptoms are more likely with higher maternal doses and longer duration of benzodiazepine use.

Patient discussion regarding benzodiazepine use during pregnancy requires conservative advice and caution [47]. It is certainly best to try to avoid benzodiazepines during pregnancy. If a patient is unable or unwilling to stop benzodiazepines because of a recurrence of disabling anxiety symptoms, she should be encouraged to use the lowest possible dose, preferably on an as-needed basis. If possible, discontinuation prior to the last 2 months of pregnancy is advisable, and the patient can restart immediately after delivery if not breast-feeding [47].

If a patient learns of a pregnancy while taking benzodiazepines, a thorough discussion and documentation of the risks and benefits of benzodiazepine use is warranted. Studies have shown that approximately 3% of all pregnancies end with an abnormal live-born infant delivered, and 3% of these infants are associated with exposure to a teratogen [47]. There is no compelling data that discontinuing benzodiazepines will decrease the 3% risk [47]. Stopping the benzodiazepine as soon as possible with a slow taper over several weeks should be encouraged.

Benzodiazepines are excreted in breast milk, and despite studies supporting a low incidence of adverse effects and toxicity, the clinician is advised to use caution and assess the risks versus benefits of exposing infants to benzodiazepines in breast milk [47].

Highlights of Benzodiazepine Use in Anxiety Disorders [Adapted from refs. 2, 47, 48, 54]

- Selective serotonin reuptake inhibitors are the preferred treatment for anxiety disorders, but benzodiazepines are commonly used to treat anxiety and anxiety disorders, despite concerns about the risk of abuse and dependence.
- Benzodiazepines have a quicker onset of action than antidepressants and are well tolerated. They can also be used on an as-needed (prn) basis.
- Benzodiazepines are useful as primary and adjunctive therapy to antidepressants for the treatment of anxiety and anxiety disorders.
- Patients treated with benzodiazepines maintain benefits over time, and according to most studies, the doses remain the same or decrease for the majority of patients.
- Appropriate prescribing of benzodiazepines requires a careful evaluation of the patient including distinguishing situational anxiety from anxiety disorders such as generalized anxiety and panic disorder.
- Discussing benzodiazepine therapy with the patient, including expected benefits, common side effects, and potential risks, can help the patient feel more comfortable and facilitates compliance with treatment.
- Patients should be warned about common side effects such as potential sedation and psychomotor impairment, as well as the issue of physical dependence and the need to taper when the drug is discontinued after longer-term use. Caution the patient about operating machinery or dangerous appliances (including driving) as well as performing skilled tasks while taking benzodiazepines, especially early in treatment. Document the information in the patient's chart.
- The clinician should advise the patient to avoid using alcohol and other sedating medications while taking benzodiazepines.
- When considering benzodiazepine therapy for elderly patients or patients with a current or lifetime history of substance abuse or dependence, the practitioner must be very cautious and thoroughly evaluate and discuss the risks and benefits with thorough documentation.
- When prescribing benzodiazepines, use the lowest effective dose. Understand physical dependence and use effective strategies for minimizing discontinuation symptoms.

- Patients with anxiety disorders who are treated with benzo-diazepines should not be viewed as drug seekers. Without a history of substance abuse, there is little liability for abuse of benzodiazepines by patients. The practitioner must reevaluate the need for benzodiazepine treatment intermittently, using good clinical judgment and attempting to taper and discontinue when possible.
- Patients who have taken benzodiazepines for many years, have a good therapeutic response, and have no evidence for misuse or abuse may be allowed to continue their medication if necessary with proper follow-up. It is generally not clinically wise to switch medications in stable, comfortable patients just for the sake of removing the benzodiazepine.

Azapirones: Buspirone

Buspirone (BuSpar) is a member of the azapirone class of medications and was the first available nonsedative, nonbenzodiazepine [1,3]. Many clinicians view it as a relatively weak anxiolytic and its efficacy has been questioned. Buspirone resembles an antipsychotic chemically more than it does any previously developed antianxiety medication or antidepressant [55]. Large doses showed insignificant beneficial effects in a phase II clinical trial of patients with schizophrenia [55]. Based on several controlled trials which have shown buspirone to be effective, it was marketed in 1986 for the treatment of GAD (Table 4.34) [3,55]. Studies of older medications such as buspirone apparently focused on safety originally, and data on efficacy (a later requirement) were not documented using current randomized controlled trials standards [55]. Many of the early buspirone studies were performed before publication of the *Diagnostic and Statistical Manual of Mental Disorders,* 3rd edition revised (DSM-III-R) when the definition of GAD was different and many of the subjects may not have had an anxiety disorder as chronic as GAD [14].

TABLE 4.34. Buspirone (BuSpar) use in anxiety disorders

- Generalized anxiety disorder (GAD)*
- Anxiety accompanying various chronic medical disorders
- Some evidence of usefulness as adjunct to antidepressants in treatment of other anxiety disorders: OCD, PTSD, social anxiety disorder

*U.S Food and Drug Administration (FDA) indication.
OCD, obsessive-compulsive disorder; PTSD, posttraumatic stress disorder.
Adapted from refs. [3], [20], [55].

Action

The antianxiety effect of buspirone is believed to occur through its action as a full agonist at presynaptic serotonin-1A receptors and a partial agonist at postsynaptic serotonin receptors [3,55]. Function at the presynaptic receptors inhibits neuronal firing and decreases serotonin synthesis [3,55]. This action is thought to account for its antianxiety activity. Buspirone acts as an agonist with a serotonin deficit but serves as an antagonist with functional serotonin excess [55].

Buspirone may be a dopamine-2 (D2) presynaptic autoreceptor antagonist, postsynaptic D2 receptor blocker, and a dopamine agonist, but the effects are not clearly understood. The major area of benzodiazepine action (benzodiazepine-GABA-chloride complex) is not affected by buspirone, although it has been shown to enhance benzodiazepine binding [55]. Buspirone may contribute to GABA anxiolytic action by indirect effects [3]. Benzodiazepine withdrawal symptoms are not affected by buspirone.

The effect of medications on cognition and psychomotor performance is very important especially in certain patients, such as the elderly. Buspirone and benzodiazepines effectively reduce cognitive (psychic) symptoms equally [3], and buspirone may have an advantage over benzodiazepines in GAD where optimum alertness and motor performance are necessary [21,55]. Buspirone may be less helpful in reducing the somatic symptoms of anxiety than benzodiazepines. Some clinicians feel buspirone is less effective in patients who have taken benzodiazepines [55].

Pharmacokinetics

Buspirone is rapidly and almost completely absorbed and undergoes extensive first-pass metabolism. Buspirone has a short half-life and is approximately 95% protein bound. It may displace less tightly protein-bound drugs, but does not appear to displace other tightly protein-bound drugs [3]. Taken with food, the absorption is delayed, and results in increased systemic blood levels of unchanged buspirone [3]. There is no evidence for differences in efficacy or adverse effects of buspirone if taken with food. Buspirone is metabolized by the CYP3A4 liver enzyme system but it is not believed to inhibit any CYP enzymes (Table 4.35) [3,55].

Buspirone has two major metabolites. The active metabolite 1-pyrimidinylpiperazine (1-PP) lacks serotonergic effects but may block α_2-noradrenergic receptors. It may cause an increase in locus ceruleus neuronal activity and increased 3-methoxy-4-hydroxyphenylglycol (MHPG) production [3,55].

TABLE 4.35. Buspirone and CYP enzyme system

Generic (trade)	CYP1A2	CYP2C9	CYP2C19	CYP2D6	CYP3A4
Buspirone (BuSpar)					s

s, substrate.
Adapted from refs. [3] and [55].

TABLE 4.36. Buspirone dosage and half-life

Generic (trade)	Indication	Starting dose*	Usual daily dose	Half-life (hours) [active metabolite]
Buspirone (BuSpar)	GAD	7.5 mg bid	30–60 mg	2–11 [6]

*Example: start 7.5 mg bid × 1 wk; increase dose by 5 mg/d q2–3d; max: 60 mg/d.
GAD, generalized anxiety disorder.
Adapted from refs. [2], [3], and [20].

TABLE 4.37. Adverse effects of buspirone

• Dizziness	• Light-headedness
• Nausea	• Agitation
• Headache	• Disturbed dreams
• Nervousness	• Akathisia (rare)

Adapted from refs. [3] and [55].

Clinical Use

Buspirone should be started at a lower dose and titrated upward to a range of 30 to 60 mg per day (Table 4.36) [2,3,20]. Lower doses may be required in patients with liver or kidney impairment because of a potential prolonged half-life. It usually takes 3 to 4 weeks and sometimes several months to obtain a therapeutic effect. There is evidence to suggest that buspirone may be useful in the treatment of anxiety disorders other than GAD when used as adjuncts to antidepressants [2]. The effects of buspirone may also increase over time.

Adverse Effects

Buspirone has few, generally mild side effects. Common adverse effects include dizziness, headache, nausea, and nervousness (Table 4.37) [3,55]. Doses may need to be reduced in patients with liver or kidney disease. Drug–drug interactions may occur but are generally benign [3,55] (Table 4.38). Sedation, psychomotor performance

TABLE 4.38. Examples of buspirone–drug interactions

- Haloperidol: modest haloperidol level elevation reported
- Cyclosporin A levels may be elevated
- MAOIs: associated with blood pressure elevation
- Nordiazepam (diazepam metabolite) concentrations may be elevated
- CYP3A4 inhibitors (e.g., erythromycin, itraconazole, grapefruit juice, verapamil, diltiazem) increase buspirone plasma levels

Adapted from refs. [2], [20], and [55].

impairment, abuse, dependence, withdrawal, and lethality in over-dose are not associated with buspirone [1,55]. Buspirone is pregnancy category B. It is not for use in nursing [20].

Tricyclic Antidepressants

A major breakthrough in the classification and treatment of anxiety disorders occurred in the 1960s with the discovery that imipramine (Tofranil) prevented panic attacks [2]. Tricyclic antidepressants and heterocyclic medications were widely prescribed for anxiety disorders such as panic disorder (with/without agoraphobia) and GAD until the advent of the novel antidepressants such as the SSRIs. In the short term, TCAs appear at least equivalent to benzodiazepines, are more effective in the long term, and are particularly effective in reducing the psychic symptoms of anxiety such as dysphoria [21,56]. It appears that a more predictable antianxiety response occurs with the tertiary amine TCAs.

First-line medications for obsessive-compulsive disorder include medications with serotonin reuptake inhibition effects, including the tricyclic clomipramine (Anafranil). Clomipramine was found to have equal or greater efficacy than SSRIs in a large meta-analysis, and other direct comparison studies but has the drawback of increased anticholinergic side effects and seizure potential [19]. Tricyclic antidepressants such as imipramine have demonstrated benefit in the treatment of GAD and panic disorder [21]. The effectiveness of TCAs in treating GAD is based on retrospective studies of subjects with anxiety states similar to current criteria for GAD [4]. Studies have reported clomipramine to be effective in the treatment of panic disorder, and one study showed desipramine (Norpramin, Pertofrane) to be more effective than placebo [4]. Tricyclic antidepressants such as imipramine (Tofranil) and amitriptyline (Elavil) have been shown to be more effective than placebo in the short-term treatment of posttraumatic stress disorder symptoms in male combat veterans [21].

Pharmacokinetics

Tricyclic antidepressants are relatively rapidly absorbed in the small intestine, and peak levels occur approximately 2 to 8 hours after ingestion. They are lipophilic compounds and have a high volume of distribution throughout the body. They are highly protein bound [57]. Metabolism of TCAs begins during the first-pass effect, resulting in a reduced amount of medication entering the systemic circulation [57]. The main clearance method for TCAs is via hepatic metabolism with a small portion of drug being eliminated by the kidneys. Elimination half-lives for most TCAs are ≥24 hours.

The two main metabolic pathways in the liver are demethylation of side chains and hydroxylation of the ring structure [57]. The CYP enzyme system appears to be responsible for hydroxylation and CYP1A2, CYP3A4, and CYP2C19 appear to be involved in demethylation [57]. Most of the TCAs exhibit linear kinetics (concentration increases in proportion to dose within the therapeutic range).

Tertiary amines such as imipramine and clomipramine are more potent serotonin reuptake inhibitors, and the secondary amines such as nortriptyline (Pamelor, Aventyl) and desipramine are more potent norepinephrine reuptake inhibitors (Table 4.39) [21,57]. Tricyclic antidepressants also inhibit the reuptake of dopamine to a lesser extent. Many of the side effects of the TCAs occur as a result of the blockade of muscarinic cholinergic receptors, histamine (H1) receptors, and α_1-adrenergic receptors (Table 4.40) [21]. Tertiary amines tend to have more side effects than do secondary amines. The tertiary tricyclic compounds are demethylated to secondary amine compounds.

TABLE 4.39. Tertiary and secondary amine TCAs

Tertiary
- Imipramine (Tofranil)
- Amitriptyline (Elavil)
- Clomipramine (Anafranil)
- Trimipramine (Surmontil)
- Doxepin (Sinequan)

Secondary
- Desipramine (Norpramin, Pertofrane)
- Nortriptyline (Pamelor, Aventyl)
- Protriptyline (Vivactil)

Adapted from refs. [21] and [57].

TABLE 4.40. TCA side effects

• Muscarinic cholinergic receptor blockade (anticholinergic effects)
• Histamine (H1) receptor blockade (sedative effects)
• α_1-adrenergic receptor blockade (orthostatic hypotension)

Adapted from ref. [21].

TABLE 4.41. Examples of TCA dosing strategies for anxicty disorders

Imipramine
• Week one: 25–50 mg/d (divided initially)
• Week two: increase to 100–150 mg as tolerated
• Week three: can increase to 225 mg/d; maximum dosage: 300 mg/d by fourth week
• Lower starting doses (50% lower) and slower titration for some patients (significant anxiety, panic, tendency to be sensitive to side effects, elderly, cardiovascular/liver disease)

Clomipramine
• Initial: 25 mg/d
• Increase within 2 weeks to 100 mg/d as tolerated
• Increase further as necessary/tolerated over several weeks to a max of 250 mg/d
• Do not exceed 250 mg/d due to increased seizure risk with higher dosages

Nortriptyline
• Week one: 25 mg/d
• Increase to 75 mg/d over 1–2 weeks as tolerated
• Maximum dosage: 150 mg/d
• Lower starting doses (50% lower) and slower titration for some patients (significant anxiety, panic, tendency to be sensitive to side effects, elderly, cardiovascular/liver disease)

Adapted from refs. [4], [20], and [21].

Clinical Use

Initial doses of TCAs for patients with significant anxiety or panic should be at least 50% lower than regular dosing for depression. If TCAs are prescribed for the elderly or patients with hepatic or cardiovascular disease, lower doses should be used. Examples of dosing strategies are listed in Table 4.41 [4,20,21].

Adverse Effects and Risks

Examples of TCA side effects are listed in Table 4.42 [21]. The blockade of muscarinic receptors by TCAs results in anticholinergic side effects. Anticholinergic side effects and overdose effects are listed

TABLE 4.42. Side effects of TCAs

Anticholinergic	Weight gain	Neurological effects
Sedation	Increased sweating	Allergic reactions
Cardiac effects	Sexual dysfunction	Potentially lethal in overdose

Adapted from ref. [21].

TABLE 4.43. TCA anticholinergic side effects

Dry mouth	Tachycardia
Constipation	Cognitive impairment (especially elderly)
Blurred vision	Confusion (especially elderly)
Urinary retention (serious)	Exacerbation of narrow angle glaucoma (serious)

Adapted from ref. [21].

TABLE 4.44. Symptoms of anticholinergic overdose

- Delirium
- Agitation
- Supraventricular arrhythmias
- Hallucinations
- Severe hypertension
- Seizures

Adapted from ref. [21].

in Tables 4.43 and 4.44 [21]. Extra caution must be exercised when prescribing antidepressants with anticholinergic side effects to patients with certain medical conditions such as cognitive impairment, narrow-angle glaucoma, and prostatic hypertrophy. Treatment of anticholinergic side effects includes dosage reduction, using an alternative antidepressant with fewer anticholinergic side effects, and addition of a cholinergic medication such as bethanechol [21].

Sedation side effects are related to histamine receptor binding. Cardiovascular effects of TCAs include orthostatic hypotension and conduction delay (Tables 4.45 and 4.46) [21,57]. Nortriptyline is the TCA least likely to cause orthostatic hypotension [21]. Clomipramine is associated with a dose-related risk of seizures, but the lowering of the seizure threshold with therapeutic doses of other TCAs is controversial [21].

Patients with ischemic heart disease are at increased risk for sudden death from TCA use. Tricyclic antidepressants are potentially lethal in overdose, primarily secondary to cardiac arrhythmia [57]. Ten times the total daily dose of a TCA can be fatal [57]. Tricyclic

TABLE 4.45. Cardiovascular side effects of TCAs

- Orthostatic hypotension
- Cardiac conduction delays
- Increased heart rate
- Arrhythmias (e.g., at toxic levels)

Adapted from ref. [21].

TABLE 4.46. Summary of TCA use and clinical implications of cardiac effects

- Adults without cardiac disease: orthostatic hypotension may occur; conduction problem not likely
- Patients with preexisting conduction delay: may cause heart block
- Patients with ischemic heart disease: continued use increases heart work, reduces heart rate variability, possibly increases sudden death risk
- Overdose: cardiac arrhythmia most common cause of death

Adapted from ref. [57].

TABLE 4.47. Examples of pharmacokinetic effects of TCAs used with other medications

Enzyme inhibition
- 2D6 inhibition: quinidine, fluoxetine, bupropion, some antipsychotics raise TCA levels
- 1A2 inhibition: TCAs may increase warfarin levels

Enzyme induction
- 3A4 induction: barbiturates, carbamazepine, phenytoin may lower TCA concentrations
- 1A2 induction: nicotine may lower TCA concentrations

Adapted from ref. [57].

antidepressants do not reduce cardiac contractility or output, however [57].

Metabolism and Drug Interactions

Tricyclic antidepressants (TCAs) are metabolized by the liver. Plasma TCA levels may be altered by drugs that inhibit or induce liver microsomal enzymes [21]. Cytochrome P-450 2D6 inhibitors may cause dangerously high levels of TCAs.

Examples of pharmacokinetic and pharmacodynamic effects that may occur due to the interaction of TCAs and other medications are included in Tables 4.47 and 4.48 [57].

TABLE 4.48. Examples of pharmacodynamic effects of TCAs used with other medications

- TCAs with MAOIs: potentially fatal hypertensive reaction
- TCAs with benzodiazepines: increased sedation
- TCAs with quinidine: potentially additive effects

Adapted from ref. [57].

Pregnancy and Lactation

There is a long history of TCA use without birth defects being observed [57]. The clinician must carefully discuss and document the risks and benefits of treating a woman with TCAs during pregnancy. If TCAs are used during pregnancy, dosage adjustments due to pregnancy metabolic changes may be necessary [57]. Neonatal drug withdrawal following delivery can occur, and so if used, TCAs should be discontinued about 1 week prior to delivery if possible [57]. Tricyclic antidepressants are excreted in breast milk, but the quantities delivered are small and usually undetectable in the milk [57]. According to the PDR, the safety in pregnancy and nursing for desipramine, nortriptyline, doxepin, and protriptyline is not known. Clomipramine and amitriptyline are pregnancy category C and not for use in nursing. Trimipramine is pregnancy category C and safety in nursing are not known. Safety for imipramine in pregnancy is not known and it is not for use in nursing [20].

Monoamine Oxidase Inhibitors

The effectiveness of MAOIs as antidepressants was first identified in the late 1950s [58]. Iproniazid, an antituberculosis medication, was noted to have mood-elevating properties and it was determined that it potently inhibited central nervous system (CNS) monoamine oxidase enzymes [58,59]. It was soon discovered that iproniazid caused hepatotoxicity, and it was removed from the market. Other MAOIs were introduced as antidepressants in the 1960s including phenelzine (Nardil) and tranylcypromine (Parnate) (Table 4.49) [20,21,59].

There are two monoamine oxidase (MAO) isoenzymes in the CNS: MAO-A and MAO-B. Dopamine, norepinephrine, serotonin, and tyramine are substrates for MAO-A, and dopamine, tyramine, and phenylethylamine are substrates for MAO-B [21]. The MAOIs block the inactivation of norepinephrine, serotonin, dopamine, and tyramine, resulting in an increase in the amount of transmitter available for release from the synapse [21]. The early MAOIs are not specific for any MAO enzyme subtype and are irreversible

TABLE 4.49. Monoamine oxide inhibitors

Generic (trade)	Start dose	Therapeutic dose*	Selectivity
Phenelzine (Nardil)	15 mg	15–90 mg/d	Nonselective
Tranylcypromine (Parnate)	10 mg	20–60 mg/d	Nonselective

*Dose 2 to 3 times/day.
Adapted from refs. [20], [21], and [59].

inhibitors. L-deprenyl (Selegiline) is a newer MAOI that is a MAO-B inhibitor. Moclobemide is a reversible MAO-A inhibitor that is not available in the U.S. [59].

Many practitioners avoid MAOI use because of the side effects, strict dietary monitoring requirements, and potential for a hypertensive crisis. The potential for serious food and drug interactions is certainly a concern. The hypertensive crisis associated with MAOIs is often referred to as the "cheese reaction." This can occur when food, tyramine-containing beverages, and other indirectly acting sympathomimetic amines are combined with MAOIs [59].

Use in Anxiety Disorders

The MAOIs are useful in a wide range of psychiatric disorders including anxiety disorders. Studies have shown MAOIs effective in treating panic disorder, generalized social anxiety, and posttraumatic stress disorder, and they may be effective in treating obsessive-compulsive disorder and GAD [2,58].

The overall role of MAOIs is small, with the increasing utilization of newer, safer, user-friendly medications for the management of anxiety disorders. Practitioners who choose to prescribe MAOIs (e.g., for treatment resistance) must familiarize themselves with the medication prescribing information as well as the current recommendations for dietary modification. Patients treated with MAOIs must follow a special very low tyramine diet to reduce the risk of a hypertensive crisis, which can include headache and stroke.

Side Effects and Interactions

The MAOIs generally cause more frequent or severe side effects than other antidepressants [59]. Side effects include postural hypotension, weight gain, and insomnia (Table 4.50) [2,21,56,59]. Important MAOI drug–drug interactions include TCAs, SSRIs, over-the-counter (OTC) medications such as cough syrups containing sympathomimetic agents, and meperidine (Table 4.51) [59]. The practitioner must always be cognizant of potential

TABLE 4.50. Side effects of MAOIs

Orthostatic hypotension	Myoclonic jerks	Paresthesia
Headache	Liver enzyme elevation	Withdrawal symptoms
Insomnia/somnolence	Carbohydrate craving	Syndrome of inappropriate antidiuretic hormone secretion
Weight gain	Pyridoxine deficiency	
Sexual dysfunction	Hypomania	
Peripheral edema	Disorientation	Restlessness
Anticholinergic	Hypoglycemia	Agitation
Nausea	Peripheral neuropathy (rare)	
Weakness	Speech blockage (rare)	

Adapted from refs. [2], [21], [56], and [59].

TABLE 4.51. MAOI–drug interactions

• Other MAOIs	• Meperidine	• Oral hypoglycemics
• TCAs	• Dextromethorphan	• Carbamazepine
• SSRIs	• Direct/indirect sympathomimetics	• Cyclobenzaprine
• Stimulants	• L-tryptophan	• Tyramine (dietary)
• Buspirone	• Fenfluramine	• Barbiturates

Adapted from refs. [21] and [59].

drug interactions and dietary issues that could result in serious conditions such as serotonin syndrome or hypertensive crisis if a patient is taking an MAOI. Medical contraindications to MAOI use include pheochromocytoma, congestive heart failure (CHF), and a history of hepatic impairment. Safety in pregnancy and nursing for phenelzine and tranylcypromine is not known [20].

Hydroxyzine

Hydroxyzine (Atarax, Vistaril) is an antihistamine receptor antagonist that has been used in psychiatry for its sedative and anticholinergic effects. It has been available since the 1950s, and has been shown to be efficacious as an anxiolytic [60]. Hydroxyzine does not depress the cortex but may suppress key CNS subcortical regions [60].

The role of histamine in the pathophysiology and possibly the treatment of anxiety may be more significant than previously

TABLE 4.52. Hydroxyzine: FDA approved for anxiety indication

Generic (trade)	Common dosage	Anxiety indication
Hydroxyzine (Atarax, Vistaril)	50–100 mg tid-qid	Anxiety and tension due to psychological factors

Adapted from refs. [4], [8], and [20].

thought. Recent research showed an increased turnover of histamine in the CNS due to increased acute and chronic stress [8].

Hydroxyzine has been studied in generalized anxiety disorder and is approved by the FDA for use in anxiety and tension due to psychological factors (Table 4.52) [4,8,20].

The use of histamine (H1) receptor antagonists in psychiatry has been common for nonspecific sedation and mild hypnotic effects [8], but benzodiazepines have largely replaced these medications. Histamine (H1) antagonists may be helpful for sedation in patients with a history of alcohol and other substance abuse because of lower abuse and dependence potential compared to benzodiazepines.

Adverse Effects

The side effects of hydroxyzine include dry mouth and drowsiness. Clinically significant respiratory depression does not appear to occur at recommended doses [60]. Stupor and convulsions may occur if a patient takes dosages significantly higher than recommended [60]. Hydroxyzine HCL (Atarax) is not for use in pregnancy (especially early pregnancy) or nursing, and the safety of hydroxyzine pamoate (Vistaril) in pregnancy is unknown (contraindicated in early pregnancy) and is not for use in nursing [20].

Other Medications for Common Anxiety Disorders

Generalized Anxiety Disorder

The most commonly used medications for GAD include the antidepressants and benzodiazepines. Antidepressants include SSRIs, SNRIs, and TCAs. The azapirone buspirone has also been shown to be effective for GAD, and mirtazapine (Remeron) has been shown to benefit patients with GAD [19]. Pregabalin (Lyrica) has demonstrated efficacy in rapidly reducing anxiety in GAD [19], and tiagabine (Gabitril) may also be effective for GAD symptoms [1,12]. There is evidence to support the use of atypical antipsychotics for anxiety [19].

Social Anxiety Disorder

First-line treatment for social anxiety disorder (SAD) includes SSRIs and SNRIs. Benzodiazepines, including clonazepam (Klonopin), are effective for SAD symptoms [12,19]. The TCA imipramine and the MAOIs phenelzine (Nardil) and tranylcypromine (Parnate) have been shown to be effective treatments for SAD [7,12,19] but are used less often due to their side-effect profiles. Valproic acid (Depakote) may be an effective treatment for SAD [12]. There is evidence that augmentation with buspirone (BuSpar), levetiracetam (Keppra), gabapentin (Neurontin), tiagabine (Gabitril), and pregabalin (Lyrica) may be helpful in patients who have an inadequate response to SSRIs [19]. Beta-blockers are useful for performance anxiety but not for the generalized form of SAD.

Panic Disorder

Many antidepressants are effective in preventing panic attacks. All currently available SSRIs and the SNRI venlafaxine extended release (Effexor XR) have demonstrated effectiveness for panic disorder symptoms [19]. Benzodiazepines are also effective for the treatment of panic disorder, especially treatment-resistant cases [12]. The practitioner must keep in mind that the benzodiazepines have a potential for abuse, especially in patients with a history for substance use disorders. The TCAs and MAOIs are also effective for the treatment of panic disorder. Valproic acid (Depakote) may be useful for treatment-resistant panic disorder [2]. Buspirone has been found to be helpful as an adjunctive treatment medication [7].

Obsessive-Compulsive Disorder

First-line medications for the treatment of obsessive-compulsive disorder (OCD) include the SSRIs and the TCA clomipramine (Anafranil). Patients with a partial response to treatment may benefit from augmentation with clonazepam (Klonopin), the atypical antipsychotics such as risperidone (Risperdal), quetiapine (Seroquel), olanzapine (Zyprexa), and aripiprazole (Abilify), as well as the typical antipsychotics haloperidol (Haldol) and pimozide (Orap) [7,12,19].

Posttraumatic Stress Disorder

The SSRIs are often considered first-line medications for posttraumatic stress disorder (PTSD), followed by venlafaxine (Effexor, Effexor XR), trazodone (Desyrel), and mirtazapine (Remeron) [7,19]. Posttraumatic stress disorder has a high rate of psychiatric comorbidity, and studies have suggested that the medication choice depends on the patient's core symptoms [7]. The TCAs and

MAOIs are also efficacious [7]. The α_1-adrenergic antagonist prazosin (Minipress) may be useful for sleep-related problems such as insomnia and nightmares in patients with PTSD who are resistant to other therapies such as the SSRIs [2,19]. Anticonvulsants such as topiramate (Topamax), lamotrigine (Lamictal), and levetiracetam (Keppra), as well as guanfacine (Tenex) and clonidine (Catapres) appear promising in the treatment of PTSD symptoms [2]. Quetiapine (Seroquel) may be effective in combat-related PTSD as an adjunctive medication [12]. Baclofen (Lioresal) is effective in treating PTSD with depression and anxiety in chronic combat-related PTSD [12].

SUMMARY

Specific medications for the various anxiety disorders include SSRIs, SNRIs, benzodiazepines, buspirone, and others. Practitioners should consult current prescribing information for more detailed prescribing information such as dosage recommendations, side effects, and drug interactions. Generally, initial prescription of lower dosages is prudent to minimize side effects, but ultimately upper dosage ranges may be necessary for anxiety disorder symptom remission. A careful, thorough discussion with the patient of the anxiety disorder and the risks and benefits of treatment is important. The use of medications to treat anxiety disorders in pregnancy is a complex area, and nonpharmacologic treatment is preferable if possible. The practitioner must keep abreast of current recommendations in the literature, monitor FDA advisories, and consult with experts such as obstetricians when indicated.

The anxiety disorder chapters discuss treatment recommendations in further detail. Remission of symptoms, with a return to appropriate function and a good quality of life, is a treatment goal. Working closely with the patient with proper follow-up monitoring is vital for reaching this goal.

References

1. Nemeroff CB. Anxiolytics: past, present, and future agents. J Clin Psychiatry 2003;64 (suppl 3):3–6.
2. Stein MB. Anxiety disorders: somatic treatment. In: Sadock BJ, Sadock VA, eds. Kaplan and Sadock's Comprehensive Textbook of Psychiatry, 8th ed., vol. 1. Philadelphia: Lippincott Williams and Wilkins, 2003:1780–1787.
3. Hudziak J, Waterman GS. Buspirone. In: Sadock BJ, Sadock VA eds. Kaplan and Sadock's Comprehensive Textbook of Psychiatry, 8th ed., vol. 2. Philadelphia: Lippincott Williams and Wilkins, 2003:2797–2801.
4. Davidson JRT, Connor KM. Treatment of anxiety disorders. In: Schatzberg AF, Nemeroff CB, eds. The American Psychiatric Publishing

Textbook of Psychopharmacology, 3rd ed. Arlington, VA: American Psychiatric Publishing, 2004:913–934.

5. Fava M. Prospective studies of adverse events related to antidepressant discontinuation. J Clin Psychiatry 2006;67(suppl 4):14–21.

6. Shelton RC. The nature of the discontinuation syndrome associated with antidepressant drugs. J Clin Psychiatry 2006;67(suppl 4):3–7.

7. Hollifield M, Mackey A, Davidson J. Integrated therapies for anxiety disorders. Psychiatr Ann 2006;36(5):329–338.

8. Nemeroff CB, Putnam JS. Antihistamines. In: Sadock BJ, Sadock VA eds. Kaplan and Sadock's Comprehensive Textbook of Psychiatry, 8th ed., vol. 2. Philadelphia: Lippincott Williams and Wilkins, 2003: 2772–2775.

9. Sussman N. General Principles of Psychopharmacology. In: Sadock BJ, Sadock VA eds. Kaplan and Sadock's Comprehensive Textbook of Psychiatry, 8th ed., vol. 2. Philadelphia: Lippincott Williams and Wilkins, 2003:2676–2699.

10. Ballenger JC. Treatment of anxiety disorders to remission. J Clin Psychiatry 2001;62 (suppl):5–9.

11. National Institute of Mental Health. Anxiety disorders. http://www.nimh.nih.gov/publicat/anxiety.cfm.

12. Waldron T, et al. Pharmacological approaches to treating anxiety disorders: new research. Psychiatric Times's Insight Into Anxiety 2004;Jan(suppl):1–8.

13. Rosenbaum JF, Tollefson GD. Fluoxetine. In: Schatzberg A F, Nemeroff CB eds. The American Psychiatric Publishing Textbook of Psychopharmacology, 3rd ed. Arlington, VA: American Psychiatric Publishing, 2004:231–246.

14. Shim J, Yonkers KA. Sertraline. In: Shatzberg AF, Nemeroff CB, eds. The American Psychiatric Publishing Textbook of Psychopharmacology, 3rd ed. Arlington, VA: American Psychiatric Publishing, 2004:247–257.

15. Herr KD, Nemeroff CB. Paroxetine. In: Schatzberg AF, Nemeroff CB, eds. The American Psychiatric Publishing Textbook of Psychopharmacology, 3rd ed. Arlington, VA: American Psychiatric Publishing, 2004:259–281.

16. Fairbanks JM, Gorman JM. Fluvoxamine. In: Schatzberg AF, Nemeroff CB, eds. The American Psychiatric Publishing Textbook of Psychopharmacology, 3rd ed. Arlington, VA: American Psychiatric Publishing, 2004:283–290.

17. Roseboom PH, Kalin NH. Citalopram and s-citalopram. In: Shatzberg AF, Nemeroff CB, eds. The American Psychiatric Publishing Textbook of Psychopharmacology, 3rd ed. Arlington, VA: American Psychiatric Publishing, 2004:291–302.

18. Kelsey JE. Selective Serotonin Reuptake Inhibitors. In: Sadock BJ, Sadock VA, eds. Kaplan and Sadock's Comprehensive Textbook of Psychiatry, 8th ed., vol. 2. Philadelphia: Lippincott Williams and Wilkins, 2005:2887–2913.

19. Davidson J. Managing anxiety disorders: psychopharmacologic treatment options. Psychiatric Times April 2006;80–83.

20. PDR Precise Prescribing Guide. Psychiatry. Issue 3. Montvale, NJ: Thompson PDR, 2006.

21. Marangell LB, Silver JM, Goff DC, Yudofsky SC. Psychopharmacology and electroconvulsive therapy. In: The American Psychiatric Publishing Textbook of Clinical Psychiatry, 4th ed., Washington, DC: American Psychiatric Publishing, 2003:1047–1083.

22. Alva G, Siegal AP, et al. Challenges in the treatment of anxiety and depression in the elderly patient. CNS News 2006;July:41–48.

23. Physicians Desk Reference, 60th ed. Montvale, NJ: Thompson PDR, 2006.

24. Hemeryck A, Belpaire FM. Selective serotonin reuptake inhibitors and cytochrome P-450 mediated drug-drug interactions: an update. Curr Drug Metab 2002;3:13–37.

25. DeBattista C, Schatzberg AF. 2003 psychotropic dosing and monitoring guidelines. Prim Psychiatry 2003;July:80–96.

26. DeVane CL. Living with an ambiguity in clinical practice: antidepressant drug-drug interactions. Insights into Depression and Anxiety, Supplement to Psychiatric Times 2006;Feb:1–8.

27. Mrazek DA, Smoller, de Leon J. Incorporating pharmacogenetics into clinical practice: reality of a new tool in psychiatry. Roundtable monograph supplement. CNS Spect 2006;11(3, suppl 3):1–13.

28. Venkatakrishnan K, Shader RI, von Moltke LL, Greenblatt DJ. Drug interactions in psychopharmacology. In: Shader RI, ed. Manual of Psychiatric Therapeutics, 3rd ed. Philadelphia: Lippincott Williams & Wilkins, 2003:441–469.

29. Hamer AM. Optimizing treatment of depression in the elderly patient. Insights into Depression and Anxiety, Supplement to Psychiatric Times 2005;Jan:1–8.

30. Roose SP, Pollock BC, Devanand DP. Treatment during late-life. In: Schatzberg AF, Nemeroff CB, eds. The American Psychiatric Publishing Textbook of Psychopharmacology, 3rd ed. Arlington, VA: American Psychiatric Publishing, 2004:1083–1091.

31. Cytochrome P450 drug-interaction table. http://medicine.iupui.edu/flockhart/.

32. Shelton RC, Lester N. Selective serotonin reuptake inhibitors and newer antidepressants. In: Stein DJ, Kupfer DJ, Schatzberg AF, eds. The American Psychiatric Publishing Textbook of Mood Disorders, 1st ed. Arlington, VA: American Psychiatric Publishing, 2006:263–280.

33. Clayton AH, Montejo AL. Major depressive disorder, antidepressants, and sexual dysfunction. J Clin Psychiatry 2006;67(suppl 6):33–37.

34. Newport DJ, Fisher A, Graybeal S, Stowe ZN. Psychopharmacology during pregnancy and lactation. In: Schatzberg AF, Nemeroff CB, eds. The American Psychiatric Publishing Textbook of Psychopharmacology, 3rd ed. Arlington, VA: American Psychiatric Publishing, 2004:1109–1136.

35. Pies R. Prenatal antidepressant use: time for a pregnant pause. Psychiatric Times http://www.psychiatrictimes.com/article/showArticle/jhtml?articleId=193006232.

36. King EZ, Stowe ZN, Newport DJ. Using antidepressants during pregnancy: an update. Psychiatric Times http://psychiatrictimes.com/article/showArticle.jhtml?articleId=102202123.

37. FDA Public Health Advisory. Treatment challenges of depression in pregnancy. http://www.fda.gov/cder/drug/advisory/SSRI_PPHN200607.htm.

38. Rubinchik SM, Kablinger AS, Gargner JS. Medications for panic disorder and generalized anxiety disorder during pregnancy. Prim Care Companion J Clin Psychiatry 2005;7(3):100–105.

39. Psychiatric News. What is the evidence base for using SSRIs during pregnancy? 2006(April 21);41;8:14. http://pn.psycjiatryonline.org/cgi/content/full/41/8/14–a.

40. Hasser C, Brizendine L, Spielvogel A. SSRI use during pregnancy. Current Psychiatry 2006;5:31–40.

41. MedPage Today. Avoid Paxil in pregnancy, ACOG committee advises. http://www.medpagetoday.com/tbprint.cfm?tbid=4611.

42. Robinson DS. Psychotropic drugs and pregnancy: guidance for antidepressants. Prim Psychiatry 2005;12(6):22–23. http://www.primarypsychiatry.com/aspx/article_pf.aspx?articleid=92.

43. Stein MB, Cantrell CR, Sokol MC, Eaddy MT, Shah MB. Antidepressant adherence and medical resource use among managed care patients with anxiety disorders. Psychiatr Serv 2006;57;5:673–680.

44. Thase ME, Sloan DME. Venlafaxine. In: Schatzberg AF, Nemeroff CB, eds. The American Psychiatric Publishing Textbook of Psychopharmacology, 3rd ed. Arlington, VA: American Psychiatric Publishing, 2004:349–360.

45. Delgado PL. How antidepressants help depression: mechanisms of action and clinical response. J Clin Psychiatry 2004;65(suppl 4):25–30.

46. Greden JF. Duloxetine and milnacipran. In: Schatzberg AF, Nemeroff CB, eds. The American Psychiatric Publishing Textbook of Psychopharmacology, 3rd ed. Arlington, VA: American Psychiatric Publishing, 2004:361–370.

47. Raj A, Sheehan D. Benzodiazepines. In: Schatzberg AF, Nemeroff CB, eds. The American Psychiatric Publishing Textbook of Psychopharmacology, 3rd ed. Arlington, VA: American Psychiatric Publishing, 2004:371–380.

48. Rosenbaum JF, chair. Utilizing benzodiazepines in clinical practice: an evidence based discussion [academic highlights]. J Clin Psychiatry 2004;65:1565–1574.

49. Feldman MD. Managing psychiatric disorders in primary care: 2. Anxiety. Hosp Pract 2000;35(7):77–84.

50. Lydiard RB. The role of GABA in anxiety disorders. J Clin Psychiatry 2003;64(suppl 3):21–27.

51. Gorman JM. New molecular targets for antianxiety interventions. J Clin Psychiatry 2003;64(suppl 3):28–35.

52. Stewart SA. The effects of benzodiazepines on cognition. J Clin Psychiatry 2005;66(suppl 2):9–13.

53. Tinsley JA. Drug abuse. In: Rakel RE, Bope ET, eds. Conn's Current Therapy, 58th ed. Philadelphia: Saunders, 2006:1344–1345.

54. Rosenbaum JF. Attitudes towards benzodiazepines over the years. J Clin Psychiatry 2005;66(suppl 2):4–8.

55. Ninan PT, Muntasser S. Buspirone and gepirone. In: Schatzberg AF, Nemeroff CB, eds. The American Psychiatric Publishing Textbook of Psychopharmacology, 3rd ed. Arlington, VA: American Psychiatric Publishing, 2004:391–404.

56. Feighner JP. Overview of antidepressants currently used to treat anxiety disorders. J Clin Psychiatry 1999;60(suppl 22):18–22.

57. Nelson JC. Tricyclic and tetracyclic drugs. In: Schatzberg AF, Nemeroff CB, eds. The American Psychiatric Publishing Textbook of Psychopharmacology, 3rd ed. Arlington, VA: American Psychiatric Publishing, 2004:207–230.

58. Krishnan KRR. Monoamine oxidase inhibitors. In: Schatzberg AF, Nemeroff CB, eds. The American Psychiatric Publishing Textbook of Psychopharmacology, 3rd ed. Arlington, VA: American Psychiatric Publishing, 2004:303–314.

59. Patkar AA, Pae C-U, Masand PS. Transdermal selegiline: a new generation of monoamine oxidase inhibitors. CNS Spectr 2006;11:363–375.

60. Hauser L, Anupindi R, Moore W. Hydroxyzine for the treatment of acute opioid withdrawal: a 20-year clinical experience. Resident and Staff Physician 2006;52:24–30.

5
Psychotherapy

Kevin T. Larkin

Given the significant documented prevalence of patients with diagnosable anxiety disorders who present to primary care medical clinics [1], physicians and other primary care practitioners frequently are called on to make recommendations regarding the effective treatment for these conditions. Health care professionals in this role have two general treatment approaches available to recommend: pharmacological approaches, which are discussed in Chapter 4, and psychotherapeutic approaches, which are discussed in this chapter. Because primary care practitioners receive significantly greater exposure to pharmacology and its clinical applications than psychotherapy during training, it is not surprising that they are much more confident in making pharmacological treatment recommendations than making recommendations for psychotherapy. However, recommending psychotherapy for treating anxiety disorders should not be overlooked, as numerous psychotherapeutic approaches have convincing therapeutic efficacy, with solid long-term follow-up data, for treating each of the anxiety disorders.

Although most primary care practitioners are not trained to carry out psychotherapy, they are capable of identifying and diagnosing anxiety disorders, assessing the disruption these disorders have on their patient's lives, and referring patients to qualified psychologists for therapy. Unfortunately, not all psychologists and other therapists employ treatment strategies known to be efficacious in treating anxiety disorders, and it is important for primary care practitioners to establish a network of referral sources that are trained in evidence-based interventions for anxiety disorders. This chapter discusses numerous psychotherapeutic approaches that have been employed with patients diagnosed with anxiety disorders, and considers empirical evidence supporting their use. Armed with this information, primary care practitioners will be better equipped to make referrals to the most qualified therapists and to support the ongoing therapeutic efforts being guided by these mental health professionals. Additionally, specific suggestions are provided pertaining to ways in which primary care providers can support the therapeutic endeavors of their patients who pursue psychotherapeutic avenues of intervention.

PSYCHOTHERAPEUTIC APPROACHES

Although countless specific psychotherapeutic approaches exist, they can generally be categorized into four predominant types: insight oriented, person centered, behavioral, and cognitive. The following subsections briefly describe each approach and provide an overview of the empirical evidence associated with the efficacy of the approach for treating anxiety disorders.

Insight-Oriented Psychotherapy

Stemming from the psychoanalytic tradition espoused by Sigmund Freud, insight-oriented therapy approaches are based on the belief that the root of anxiety disorders lies in early childhood experiences in which unconscious hedonic desires come into conflict with conventional social expectations that inhibit their expression. Failure of the developing personality to resolve these conflicts results in sustained problems with anxiety that reemerge periodically throughout life in various manifestations that vary from patient to patient (e.g., panic attacks, generalized anxiety, phobias, and compulsive rituals). Treatment, accordingly, involves gaining insight into these often well-hidden and defended conflicts through psychoanalytic treatment approaches designed to bring historic information into current awareness. Current forms of insight-oriented therapies are less steeped in the psychoanalytic tradition, but still place the primary emphasis on gaining insight into events of historic importance (e.g., trauma) and the role they play in a patient's constellation of presenting symptoms.

Person-Centered Psychotherapy

Person-centered therapeutic approaches are based on the work of humanistic personality theorists who focused on the importance of basic human worth and the innate drives for self-improvement that all humans share. Recognizing that these drives for improvement become thwarted by various types of interactions with others in our environments that create a variety of emotional responses including anxiety, sadness, and anger, Carl Rogers [2] constructed a form of therapy termed client-centered therapy. In his approach, therapy consisted of exposing the client to a genuine interaction with a nonjudgmental therapist to permit the re-centering of self-determination and letting go of expectations that others have of the client. Client-centered therapists are never confrontational and the focus of therapy is on developing and maintaining the nonjudgmental nature of the current therapeutic relationship, which serves as the foundation for anxiety reduction.

Behavior Therapy

Behavior therapy, introduced in the 1950s by Joseph Wolpe [3], among others, refers to a set of therapeutic interventions based on documented behavioral learning principles observed in laboratory-based psychological research, including the principles of classical (Pavlovian) and operant conditioning. In contrast to insight-oriented and person-centered approaches, behavioral treatment strategies are primarily focused on altering patterns of current environment-behavior relations that maintain anxiety disorders rather than uncovering historic sources of anxiety. Through the acquisition of improved anxiety management skills (e.g., relaxation strategies), patients are guided to confront situations that have previously elicited anxiety responses, commonly using a gradual approach. Various forms of behavior therapy have evolved from this tradition, including systematic desensitization (imaginally confronting a feared object) and exposure therapy (actually confronting a feared object).

Cognitive Therapy

Based on observations that patients with various forms of psychiatric disorders, including patients with anxiety disorders, displayed patterns of dysfunctional thinking, Aaron Beck [4] and Albert Ellis [5], among others, became dissatisfied with the ignorance of conscious thought processes inherent with the prevailing types of therapeutic approaches. As a result, they proposed a greater focus on identifying and correcting irrational thought patterns during therapy, a process commonly called cognitive restructuring. Although initially devised as a unique therapeutic approach, over the past few decades, cognitive restructuring strategies have been integrated with the principles of behavior change used in behavior therapy, resulting in what is commonly termed cognitive behavior therapy (CBT).

EFFICACY AND EFFECTIVENESS OF PSYCHOTHERAPY IN TREATING ANXIETY DISORDERS

Researchers examining the effect of various forms of psychotherapy for treating psychological disorders typically make a distinction between therapeutic efficacy and therapeutic effectiveness [6]. Efficacy addresses the question of "Does it work?" and effectiveness addresses the question of "How useful is it?" Highly efficacious treatments may not be effective if only a few therapists are trained to deliver them. Questions of efficacy are typically examined through well-controlled, randomized clinical trials, and questions of effectiveness are typically examined in applied settings where patient selection criteria are not as stringent and comorbidity of psychiatric diagnoses runs rampant. In general, efficacy of various psychotherapeutic approaches is established first, and questions of for whom it works best are answered through subsequent empirical work examining effectiveness in applied treatment settings.

Prior to the 1990s, there was little agreement regarding questions of therapeutic efficacy, leading some researchers to conclude that there was insufficient evidence that therapy worked at all [7] and others to conclude that all forms of therapy worked equally well [8]. This led Division 12 (Clinical Psychology) of the American Psychological Association (APA) to create the Task Force on the Promotion and Dissemination of Psychological Procedures, whose primary purpose was to examine the entire body of treatment literature and develop a strategy to ensure that evidence-based interventions were being promoted and disseminated to practicing psychologists and other therapists in the field. Not surprisingly, their first aim was to identify the various forms of therapy that were supported by solid empirical evidence. After constructing a set of criteria for evaluating the literature supporting each form of therapy, the task force assembled a list of empirically supported treatments for a number of psychological disorders, including the anxiety disorders [9]. Interventions that demonstrated superior outcome compared to a credible control condition (e.g., placebo) or another treatment on two separate occasions by independent investigators were categorized as well-established therapies, and those shown to be superior to a waiting-list control group, but yet to be examined across multiple trials, were categorized as probably efficacious interventions. A comparable rating system was employed for rating therapeutic trials conducted on children and adolescents [10]. Intervention approaches for treating anxiety disorders that met these criteria are depicted in Table 5.1 [9–11].

In the 1990s, evidence-based medicine received considerable attention from medical scientists and health care professionals. One outcome of these efforts is the regular dissemination of reports of outcomes of randomized clinical trials for a range of medical disorders, like the monthly reports of the *British Medical Journal* (BMJ) Publishing Group [11]. Using empirical evidence as a guide, this group categorizes interventions into one of six groups: beneficial, likely to be beneficial, trade-off between benefits and harms, unknown effectiveness, unlikely to be beneficial, and likely to be ineffective or harmful. Ratings from the BMJ Publishing Group for each therapeutic approach for treating anxiety disorders they have evaluated are also included in Table 5.1.

TABLE 5.1. Efficacy of psychotherapy interventions for treating anxiety disorders

Anxiety disorder diagnosis	Therapeutic approach	APA Task Force rating[1]	BMJ rating[2]
Panic disorder with agoraphobia	CBT	Well established	Beneficial
	Exposure therapy	Well established	Likely to be beneficial
Panic disorder	CBT	Well established	Beneficial
	Applied relaxation	Probably efficacious	Likely to be beneficial
	Client-centered therapy		Likely to be beneficial
	Insight-oriented therapy		Unknown effect
Specific phobia	Exposure therapy	Well established	
	Systemic desensitization	Probably efficacious	
Social phobia	CBT	Probably efficacious	
	Exposure therapy	Probably efficacious	
	Systemic desensitization	Probably efficacious	
Generalized anxiety disorder	CBT	Well established	Likely to be beneficial
	Applied relaxation	Probably efficacious	Unknown effect
Obsessive compulsive disorder	Exposure/response prevention	Well established	Beneficial
	Cognitive therapy	Probably efficacious	Beneficial
	Relapse prevention	Probably efficacious	
Posttraumatic stress disorder	Exposure therapy	Probably efficacious	
	Stress inoculation/CBT	Probably efficacious	Beneficial
	Eye movement desensitization	Probably efficacious	Beneficial
	Psychodynamic psychotherapy		Unknown effect
	Supportive psychotherapy		Unknown effect

Continued

TABLE 5.1. (continued)

Anxiety disorder diagnosis	Therapeutic approach	APA Task Force rating[1]	BMJ rating[2]
Anxiety disorders in Childhood (including separation anxiety disorder; overanxious disorder; and avoidant disorder)	CBT CBT + family anxiety training	Probably efficacious Probably efficacious	
Phobia (childhood)	Reinforced practice Participant modeling Live/filmed modeling In vivo/imaginal desensitization CBT	Well established Well established Probably efficacious Probably efficacious Probably efficacious	

[1]Categorizations based on findings from the APA Task Force [9] and Childhood Task Force [10].
[2]Categorizations based on findings from the BMJ Publishing Group [11].
Note: Blank cells indicate that no rating was made.

As depicted in Table 5.1, the vast majority of therapeutic interventions with demonstrated efficacy for treating the anxiety disorders are behavior therapy or CBT approaches. All well-established and probably efficacious therapies for anxiety disorders, as defined by the APA Task Force criteria, and all but one beneficial and likely to be beneficial therapies, as defined by the BMJ Publishing Group criteria, are behavioral or cognitive-behavioral approaches. Although insight-oriented therapeutic approaches have been used and taught for over a century now, and person-centered approaches have a considerable following, the empirical evidence supporting their use with anxiety disorders is scant. Most of the evidence supporting the use of these strategies comes from case studies, and no randomized clinical trials have been conducted examining the efficacy of them for use with any of the anxiety disorders. This is not to say that insight-oriented or person-centered approaches are not therapeutic; they simply have not been examined empirically adequately to recommend their use for treating patients with anxiety disorders.

Acknowledgment must be made of the fact that although randomized clinical trials are essential for answering questions of therapeutic *efficacy*, they are less helpful in determining which psychotherapeutic approaches are *effective* for patients presenting in primary care medical settings with various constellations of individual difference variables (e.g., demographics, comorbid medical and psychiatric disorders, presence of social support). Considerations of these individual difference variables and how they influence therapeutic outcomes has been widely discussed [12], and practicing therapists with expertise in working with patients with anxiety disorders are familiar with modifications in treatment planning that might be entertained for patients based on their unique developmental histories.

It is important to note that efficacy of CBT approaches for treating anxiety disorders parallels treatment efficacy associated with the major pharmacological approaches (e.g., selective serotonin reuptake inhibitors, benzodiazepines). Of course, significantly greater patient motivation, time, and effort are required to undergo a successful course of CBT in contrast to the effort needed to take a pill on a daily basis. This increased time commitment associated with CBT, however, has a long-term advantage over purely pharmacological approaches. Whereas patients receiving only pharmacological interventions are maintained on medications for lengthy periods of time in order to regulate symptoms of anxiety, patients completing psychotherapy can often reduce dosages or discontinue medications altogether at the completion of treatment. Although a more intensive form of treatment for anxiety disorders initially, psychotherapy is often a more cost beneficial approach in the long run [13].

COGNITIVE BEHAVIOR THERAPY APPROACH
FOR TREATING ANXIETY DISORDERS

Given the current state of the empirical literature regarding psychotherapeutic approaches to treating anxiety disorders, it is clear that primary care practitioners would be on firm footing to recommend CBT for patients interested in pursuing psychotherapeutic treatment for their anxiety disorders. To orient the patient properly for CBT and increase the probability that the patient follows through with the referral to a cognitive behavior therapist, a primary care provider should understand what a course of CBT entails. With this information, primary care practitioners can make more informed referrals to qualified therapists and can better support the ongoing therapeutic endeavor. Although the specific recommended treatment course may vary from patient to patient, CBT typically involves three stages: evaluation and education, skills acquisition, and application of skills during exposure to anxiety-eliciting stimuli. A brief description of each stage follows.

Evaluation and Education

Cognitive behavior therapy begins with a comprehensive assessment of a patient's physiological, cognitive, and behavioral symptom profile. Information pertaining to specific patterns of autonomic physiological arousal is obtained, as is information pertaining to typical thought patterns associated with anxiety. For example, a patient exhibiting panic attacks might describe experiencing physiological symptoms of heart palpitations, tightness in the chest, and shortness of breath accompanied by thoughts that he or she might be dying. Obviously, the patient's negative appraisal of these physiological symptoms fuels anxiousness, often leading the patient to engage in behaviors aimed at reducing the intolerable escalating anxiety (e.g., escape from an uncomfortable situation, checking with a health care professional). During this evaluation, the cognitive behavior therapist's primary goal is to piece together the patient's reported symptoms using something called a *functional analysis of behavior*. Often, a schematic representation of the links between various environmental stimuli and the patient's specific anxiety responses, like the one depicted in Figure 5.1, can be devised, and it plays a useful role in educating the patient in how anxiety problems are acquired and maintained. As depicted in the figure, cognitive behavior therapists attempt to identify the relations between the patient's behavioral symptoms (anxiety and escape behaviors) and the contextual variables in the patient's environment, including both observable antecedents (predictable environmental cues for anxiety) and consequences of the behavioral responses (relief). By conducting a thorough functional

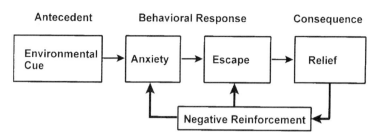

FIGURE 5.1. A functional analysis of behavior for an anxiety disorder. Specific internal and external environmental stimuli serve as antecedent cues for a patient's emotional and behavioral responses, which are followed by relief. Escape behaviors lead to anxiety reduction (relief) and maintain the anxiety disorder through negative reinforcement.

analysis of behavior, the cognitive behavior therapist can then identify the behavioral principle responsible for maintaining the anxiety symptoms. In this case, and in most cases of anxiety disorders, the principle of negative reinforcement is involved in maintaining anxiousness. Negative reinforcement is a fundamental behavioral principle in which a sequence of behaviors is maintained or increases in strength when it is followed by the removal of an undesirable state or environmental stimulus. In cases of anxiety disorders, removal of the undesirable state of anxiousness (i.e., relief) reinforces or strengthens the sequence of behaviors that preceded it, resulting in increased anxiousness in the future as well as an increased propensity for escape behaviors.

Once factors contributing to a patient's problems with anxiety have been elucidated through the functional analysis of behavior, this same model serves as a very useful tool in educating the patient about the physiological, cognitive, and behavioral components of anxiety disorders and how they are linked with one another in maladaptive ways to interfere with one's quality of life. The model depicted in the figure also serves as a useful tool for introducing the CBT treatment approach that involves acquiring anxiety management skills as well as removing escape behaviors responsible for maintaining the anxiety problem.

Skills Acquisition
Once the patient understands and chooses to participate in CBT, the next phase of treatment involves learning anxiety management skills, including both skills aimed at regulating physiological arousal and skills aimed at identifying and challenging maladaptive anxious thoughts. Although many different strategies

can be used to improve one's ability to regulate physiological arousal, the most common techniques employed in CBT include diaphragmatic breathing training, progressive muscle relaxation, guided imagery, and other forms of meditation. Regarding strategies for reducing maladaptive thoughts, several methods of cognitive restructuring are taught, including disputing irrational thoughts, challenging maladaptive patterns of thinking (e.g., catastrophic thinking), and training in self-instructional thinking. Typically, most patients with anxiety disorders emerge from this phase of treatment equipped with an array of skills for regulating physiological arousal and altering negative thought processes.

It must be noted that not all forms of behavior therapy include training in anxiety management skills, as some therapists proceed directly from the evaluation and education phase to the exposure phase of treatment. For example, exposure and response prevention therapy for obsessive-compulsive disorder does not typically involve learning skills in anxiety management prior to exposing the patient to anxiety-eliciting stimuli. In fact, acquisition of anxiety management skills while treating obsessive-compulsive conditions may not contribute to positive treatment outcomes, and in some cases may hinder progress in treatment. The majority of CBT approaches for treating anxiety disorders, however, involve acquiring a range of anxiety management skills prior to engaging in the final phase of treatment, exposure therapy.

Exposure Therapy
Through patient education it becomes quickly apparent to anxiety disorder patients engaged in CBT that they need to learn to confront anxiety rather than escape or avoid anxiety-eliciting situations in order to eliminate the negative reinforcement cycle that maintains the anxious condition. All effective forms of CBT employ some form of exposure to anxiety-eliciting stimuli, and it may be considered the critical element of therapy that results in positive outcomes. There are two general strategies for exposing patients to anxious stimuli: direct exposure (or flooding) and graduated exposure (or desensitization). Using the flooding approach, patients contact their most feared situation directly until their anxiety response habituates. This approach is highly effective and works relatively quickly, but is not too comfortable for the patient who has to endure a period of high anxiety to achieve the desired effect. Using the desensitization approach, patients practice anxiety management skills in low anxious situations first, building confidence to move on to handling moderately anxious situations and eventually high

anxious situations. This approach is also quite effective and has the added benefit that extreme anxiety is never really experienced, but therapy takes a good bit longer to achieve a comparable effect to that of the direct exposure approach. Using either approach, repeated exposure to the feared stimuli or situation results in breaking the chain of negative reinforcement that is maintaining the patient's anxiety symptoms, and the symptoms dissipate.

The actual structure of exposure therapy varies from patient to patient depending on the nature of his or her anxiety disorder. For many patients, exposure therapy can be conducted in vivo: patients with height phobia are exposed to climbing ladders, patients with social phobia are exposed to interactions with strangers, patients with posttraumatic stress disorder are exposed to the location of the traumatic event, and patients with obsessive-compulsive disorder are asked to touch items they view as contaminated. In some cases, however, in vivo exposure is not possible and imaginal exposure is used instead. For example, the cost of making repeated trips via airplane to overcome a flight phobia may prohibit frequent in vivo exposure from being used. The technology of virtual reality has also been employed for purposes of conducting exposure therapy for situations that are difficult to construct [14]. Finally, for some anxiety disorders, the feared stimuli to which the patient is exposed is an internal sensation. For example, patients with panic disorder are typically fearful of autonomic nervous system symptoms associated with having a panic attack; exposure therapy for these patients involves exposing them to bodily sensations like a racing heart (by running in place) or shortness of breath (by breathing through a straw).

COLLABORATION BETWEEN PRIMARY CARE PRACTITIONERS AND PSYCHOTHERAPISTS

For the most part, psychotherapeutic interventions of patients with anxiety disorders are conducted by clinical psychologists or other therapists working within primary medical care settings or in local mental health practice locations, although training primary care practitioners, including physicians, in CBT has been advocated [15,16]. Primary care practitioners need to know how to access their local network of therapists easily and how to collaborate with them to optimize patient care. There are several aspects to developing and maintaining productive collaborations with psychologists and other therapists that are important for primary care practitioners to consider, including handling the referral with care, managing medication, and monitoring the ongoing therapeutic process.

Making the Referral

Many patients with anxiety disorders present to primary care practitioners rather than mental health specialists because they believe the anxiety sensations they are experiencing are symptoms of an underlying medical disorder. No doubt, many patients with actual medical disorders present to their primary care practitioners with the same constellation of symptoms that patients with anxiety disorders exhibit. These patients can be sensitive to any consideration by their primary care providers that their symptoms are psychological in origin, and certainly they do not want to hear "it's all in your head." In establishing a referral for psychotherapy, it is important for the primary care practitioner to acknowledge the physical nature of their symptoms, while providing some education about how the mind and the body are linked. If well done, referrals can be a source of comfort for patients who can be relieved that their symptoms are not life threatening and that there are effective treatments for their problems with anxiety.

Although this may seem obvious, primary care practitioners should develop a network of psychologists or other therapists who are trained to implement psychotherapeutic interventions with known efficacy and effectiveness. Unfortunately, this is often easier said than done, as therapists with expertise in treating anxiety disorders are often in short supply and congregated in communities with larger populations [17]. At the present time, an optimal network of psychological service providers should be well versed in the delivery of CBT. However, it is important for primary care practitioners to maintain some familiarity with the psychological treatment literature as new discoveries are made regularly regarding alternative treatment approaches.

With the increased presence of behavioral health care clinicians in primary care medical settings, an optimum arrangement is to refer patients diagnosed with anxiety disorders to a clinical psychologist or therapist working within the medical clinic. Referrals to therapists on staff do not require the patient to enter a new health care environment for treatment, and communication between primary care practitioner and therapist is optimized if they are charting on the same medical record.

Medication Management

Many patients with anxiety disorders pursue treatment using both pharmacological and psychotherapeutic approaches. As such, primary care practitioners often find themselves in the role of managing psychopharmacological medications concurrent with the patient's participation in psychotherapy. This is not a problem as long as there is a solid collaboration between the primary care practitioner and the treating therapist. For a primary care provider who is well informed regarding the patients' progress in therapy, medication dosages would not be adjusted when the patient's anxiety levels predictably increased during the exposure phase of treatment. In contrast, uninformed primary care providers might respond to their patient's reports of increased anxiety during the exposure phase of treatment by unnecessarily increasing the dosage of an anxiolytic agent.

For most therapists, psychotherapy for anxiety disorders can proceed effectively regardless of whether patients choose to combine therapy with pharmacological management of anxiety symptoms or whether they complete therapy without using medications. Although combined therapeutic approaches are commonly used, there are two reasons to be cautious when using a combined treatment approach. First, to fully implement CBT successfully, resulting in the patient's acquisition of a degree of personal mastery over anxiety symptoms, exposure to anxiety-eliciting situations must eventually occur in a medication-free state. If pharmacological agents are not withdrawn during psychotherapy, patients with anxiety disorders never get to fully test their newly developed anxiety management skills and learn to tolerate sensations of anxiety without the knowledge that they are taking an anxiolytic agent. Thus, among patients who elect to remain on anxiolytic medications during and following treatment with CBT, the acquired anxious response is never completely extinguished.

The second limitation of using anxiolytic agents pertains to the propensity of some primary care practitioners to prescribe them on an "as-needed" basis (prn). Although prn dosing may have its place in medicine, it almost always complicates the psychotherapeutic treatment of anxiety disorders. As expected, patients given anxiolytics, specifically benzodiazepines, on a prn basis only take them when they experience anxiety. Returning to the phenomenon of negative reinforcement depicted in Figure 5.1, it is easy to see how anxiolytic use in this manner functions as a new escape behavior that perpetuates symptoms of anxiety as well as sets the stage for potential drug dependence. This is not to say that anxiolytics are not effective tools for treating anxiety disorders; they simply should not be routinely prescribed on an as-needed basis.

Monitoring Progress in Psychotherapy

Once a patient starts psychotherapy for an anxiety disorder, it is important for primary care practitioners to monitor the patient's progress in therapy and support the therapeutic endeavor. It is counterproductive for patients to receive mixed messages from their primary care provider and therapist while undergoing treatment for an anxiety condition. If a solid collaborative relationship exists between the primary care provider and the therapist, the primary care practitioner will understand the process of psychotherapy, be aware of the patient's progress, and be able to reinforce the messages the therapist is providing to the patient. For example, during the skills acquisition phase of therapy, patient progress is enhanced when a supporting primary care practitioner encourages regular practice of anxiety management skills by the patient. In contrast, patient progress will be stifled by primary care practitioners who question the validity of various anxiety management skills that are being taught during therapy sessions.

The exposure phase of the intervention often creates the most difficulty for primary care practitioners who perceive the temporary increase in anxiety associated with confronting fearful stimuli as a sign that the intervention is not working. If this skepticism is shared with their patients, patient motivation to participate in treatment can decline and, for some patients, lead to discontinuing exposure therapy as it represents the most challenging phase of therapy for many patients. Progress during the exposure phase of CBT is enhanced when primary care practitioners acknowledge the difficulty of this stage of treatment to their patients and encourage them to adhere to the treatment. In fact, in a study of panic disorder patients conducted in an emergency room setting, brief exposure

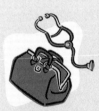

Pearls for the Practitioner

- Acknowledge the patient's experience of anxiety symptoms when considering an anxiety disorder diagnosis.
- Using the latest empirical evidence, recommend both pharmacological and CBT intervention approaches.
- Reassure the patient that effective treatments are available for his or her anxiety disorder.
- Establish a collaborative network of clinical psychologists and/or other therapists trained to conduct CBT for treating anxiety disorders.

Continued

Continued

- Monitor and support patients' progress during psychotherapy.
- Encourage acquisition and ongoing practice of anxiety management skills.
- Be aware that a patient's anxiety level sometimes increases temporarily during exposure therapy and that this is no cause for alarm.
- Never routinely prescribe anxiolytic agents on an "as-needed" basis for patients with anxiety disorders.

instructions provided by a member of the medical team were sufficient in reducing symptoms of anxiety among these patients [18].

Summary

Numerous forms of psychotherapy have been conducted on patients with anxiety disorders over the past century, including insight-oriented, person-centered, behavioral, and cognitive approaches. In general, empirical evidence has supported the use of cognitive and behavioral forms of treatment (e.g., CBT) for treating anxiety disorders much more so than insight-oriented and person-centered therapeutic approaches. Cognitive behavior therapy is an accepted treatment approach that involves conducting a thorough evaluation of a patient's specific anxiety symptoms, providing education to the patient regarding why his or her problems with anxiety are being maintained, training the patient in improved anxiety management skills, and exposing the patient to sources of anxiety in order to apply his or her newly acquired anxiety management skills. Outcome findings for CBT have been impressive, and in some cases (e.g., specific phobia, obsessive-compulsive disorder, posttraumatic stress disorder) they are the treatments of choice. Despite the empirical evidence supporting CBT as a first-line treatment for anxiety disorders, the majority of patients with anxiety disorders are offered other forms of less effective therapies [19], and the availability of CBT expertise in primary medical care settings is lacking [15,20]. Through increased collaboration between primary care practitioners and psychotherapists and the increased presence of behavioral health care providers in primary medical care settings, patients with anxiety disorders will have improved access to empirically supported treatment approaches, and their problems with anxiety will be more effectively diagnosed and treated.

References

1. Harmon JS, Rollman BL, Hanusa BH, Lenze EJ, Shear KM. Physician office visits of adults for anxiety disorders in the United States, 1985–1998. J Gen Intern Med 2002;17:165–172.
2. Rogers CR. Client-Centered Therapy. Boston: Houghton-Mifflin, 1951.
3. Wolpe J. Psychotherapy by Reciprocal Inhibition. Stanford, CA: Stanford University Press, 1958.
4. Beck AT. Cognitive Therapy and the Emotional Disorders. New York: International Universities Press, 1976.
5. Ellis A. Reason and Emotion in Psychotherapy. New York: Lyle Stuart, 1962.
6. Onken LS, Blaine JD, Battjes RJ. Behavioral therapy research: a conceptualization of a process. In: Henggeler SW & Santos AB, eds. Innovative Approaches for Difficult to Treat Populations. Washington, DC: American Psychiatric Press, 1997:477–485.
7. Eysenck HJ. The effects of psychotherapy: an evaluation. J Consult Psychol 1952;16:319–324.
8. Luborsky L, Singer B, Luborsky L. Comparative studies of psychotherapies: Is it true that "everyone has won and all must have prizes"? Arch Gen Psychiatry 1975;32:995–1008.
9. Chambless DL, Baker MJ, Baucom DH, et al. Update on empirically validated therapies, II. Clin Psychol 1998;51:3–16.
10. Ollendick TH, King NJ. Empirically supported treatments for children with phobic and anxiety disorders: current status. J Clin Child Psychol 1998;27:156–167.
11. British Medical Journal Publishing Group. Clinical Evidence Concise: The International Source of the Best Available Evidence for Effective Health Care, vol. 15. London: BMJ Publishing Group, 2006.
12. Castonguay LG, Beutler LE, eds. Principles of Therapeutic Change that Work. New York: Oxford University Press, 2006.
13. Otto MW, Pollack MH, Maki KM. Empirically supported treatments for panic disorder: costs, benefits, and stepped care. J Consult Clin Psychol 2000;68:556–563.
14. Wiederhold BK, Wiederhold MD. Virtual Reality Therapy for Anxiety Disorders: Advances in Evaluation and Treatment. Washington, DC: American Psychological Association, 2005.
15. Demertzis KH, Craske MG. Cognitive-behavioral therapy for anxiety disorders in primary care. Prim Psychiatry 2005;12:52–58.
16. Shear MK, Schulberg HC. Anxiety disorders in primary care. Bull Menninger Clin 1995;59(2A):A73–85.
17. Lader M. Treatment of anxiety. Br Med J 1994;309:321–324.
18. Swinson RP, Soulios C, Cox BJ, Kuch K. Brief treatment of emergency room patients with panic attacks. Am J Psychiatry 1992;149:944–946.
19. Goisman RM, Warshaw MG, Keller MB. Psychosocial treatment prescriptions for generalized anxiety disorder, panic disorder, and social phobia, 1991–1996. Am J Psychiatry 1999;156:1819–1821.
20. Barlow DH, Lehman CL. Advances in the psychosocial treatment of anxiety disorders. Implications for national health care. Arch Gen Psychiatry 1996;53:727–735.

6
Adjustment Disorder with Anxiety

John R. Vanin

Adjustment disorder with anxiety is not an official category of anxiety disorders in the *Diagnostic and Statistical Manual of Mental Disorders*, 4th edition, text revision (DSM-IV-TR). It is a common subthreshold disorder, however, and can be associated with significant psychopathology. It is an important disorder for the primary care practitioner to recognize and treat.

An adjustment disorder is defined as a psychological response to an identifiable psychosocial stressor [1,2]. It is a subthreshold diagnosis and it lies in a "gray" zone. The symptoms are clinically significant, develop within 3 months of a stressor's onset, and persist for no more than 6 months once the stressor is terminated. Adjustment disorder symptoms are marked by distress, or significant social, occupational, or academic dysfunctioning beyond what would be expected for a given stressor (Table 6.1) [1]. A primary care practitioner must recognize that an adjustment disorder is a residual diagnostic category describing a response to an identifiable stressor and not meeting the criteria for another major mental disorder.

Adjustment disorders are classified according to their clinical features. The predominant symptom subtypes of an adjustment disorder include anxiety, mixed anxiety and depressed mood, depressed mood, and various disturbances in conduct [1]. Despite the fact that an adjustment disorder must resolve within 6 months of a stressor's termination, symptoms may persist longer than 6 months if the stressor is chronic. Examples of situations that may result in prolonged adjustment disorder symptoms include chronic general medical conditions and persistent financial difficulties.

Adjustment disorders with anxiety symptoms may occur because of a single factor or multiple stressors. Stressors may be recurrent or continuous conditions. Examples of stressors that may cause anxiety include job difficulties, marital problems, and financial hardship (Table 6.2) [2].

Anxiety symptoms include worry, nervousness, and sleep disturbance. Some patients have a combination of anxious and depressive

TABLE 6.1. Diagnostic criteria for adjustment disorder

- Development of emotional or behavioral symptoms occurring within 3 months of an identifiable stressor's onset
- Symptoms or behaviors are clinically significant because of excessively marked distress or significant social, occupational, or academic impairment
- Symptoms do not persist for more than 6 months once the stressor or its consequences has terminated
- The stress-related symptoms do not meet the criteria for another specific Axis I mental disorder and is not an exacerbation of a preexisting Axis I or II disorder
- Symptoms are not bereavement related
- Subtypes include with anxiety, with mixed anxiety and depressed mood, with depressed mood, with disturbance of conduct, with mixed disturbance of emotions and conduct, unspecified

Adapted from ref. [1].

TABLE 6.2. Examples of stressors causing an adjustment disorder with anxiety

- Occupational, academic, social difficulties
- Marriage/divorce
- Financial hardship
- Becoming a parent
- Diagnosis of a serious medical disorder
- Retirement

Adapted from ref. [2].

symptoms. The clinician must be aware that an adjustment disorder can be diagnosed in addition to another Axis I mental disorder such as depression or an anxiety disorder.

ASSOCIATED FEATURES

Patients who suffer from an adjustment disorder may have subjective distress or functional impairment. This is often manifested as performance problems at work or school and in relationships. Adjustment disorders may be associated with suicidal behavior, excessive substance use, and somatic symptoms [1]. Strain and Newcorn cited an observation by Runeson et al. that noted in patients with an adjustment disorder, the median interval between the first communication of suicide and suicide was very short (<1 month) compared to a longer period in other mental disorders including major depression [3]. Individuals with preexisting mental disorders can also have an adjustment disorder, and adjustment disorder symptoms can complicate a general medical condition. The symptoms can be varied and triggered by stressors of any severity.

EPIDEMIOLOGY

When the practitioner makes a clinical judgment regarding a patient's response to a stressor, the cultural setting must be considered. The response and meaning of the stressors may vary across cultures [1]. Adjustment disorders occur at any age, and in adults the female to male ratio is 2:1 [3]. Prevalence rates vary widely, and community samples of children, adolescents, and the elderly describe the rate as between 2% and 8% [1,3]. In general hospital patients referred for mental health consultation, the prevalence of adjustment disorder is up to 12% [1,3]. Adjustment disorder has been diagnosed in as many as 50% in special populations of patients who have experienced specific stressors such as cardiac surgery [1,3]. Adjustment disorders are frequently diagnosed in patients after head and neck surgery and in patients with other severe medical problems such as cancer, HIV, inpatients suffering from burns, early-stage multiple sclerosis, and patients who have suffered from strokes [3]. Disadvantaged individuals may be at an increased risk for an adjustment disorder [1]. Strain and Newcorn discussed a study by Friedman et al. that found adjustment disorder was a risk factor for poor family functioning [3].

COURSE AND PROGNOSIS

The onset of an adjustment disorder is usually immediately after an acute stressor or crisis, and the duration is usually fairly brief. The disorder may persist if a stressor or its consequences persists. The primary care practitioner must evaluate for comorbid conditions such as other anxiety disorders or depression. The long-term prognosis of an adjustment disorder in adults is good overall, compared to that in younger populations [3]. Despite this statistically good prognosis, Strain and Newcorn discussed a study by Despland et al. that observed 52 patients at the end of treatment or after 3 years of treatment and found 31% had a psychiatric comorbidity, 14% had attempted suicide, 29% developed a more serious psychiatric disorder, and 23% showed an unfavorable clinical state [3]. Clinicians must consider and appropriately diagnose adjustment disorders. Even though it is considered a subthreshold diagnosis, an adjustment disorder is an important disorder to recognize and treat.

ETIOLOGY

There are many variables and modifiers regarding who will experience an adjustment disorder, but the etiology has been described as stress [3]. For example, a stressor that objectively appears major to many may have little effect on one person, but a minor stressor may be regarded as overwhelming by another individual. Strain and Newcorn also cited a study by Hamburg which described an additive effect for a recent minor stress superimposed on an underlying nonobservable major stress [3]. The practitioner may find assessing an individual's vulnerability, such as ego strength, control over stressors, timing of the stressor, support system, underlying personality disorder features, and additive effects, is helpful in determining how important a stressor is to an individual [3].

DIFFERENTIAL DIAGNOSIS

Adjustment disorder is a residual diagnostic category. The presenting symptoms are a response to an identifiable stressor and do not meet another specific Axis I mental disorder criteria [1]. Other disorders that are commonly considered in the differential disorder are listed in Table 6.3 [1].

TREATMENT

The primary treatment of adjustment disorders includes psychotherapy, education, and psychosocial interventions [1]. Table 6.4 lists different forms of talk therapy that a primary care practitioner may consider [3].

The goals of talk therapy include examining ways of reducing the stressors, coping better with stressors that cannot be reduced

TABLE 6.3. Differential diagnosis of adjustment disorder

- Acute stress disorder/posttraumatic stress disorder
- Other anxiety disorders
- Personality disorders
- Psychological factors affecting a medical condition
- Bereavement
- Direct physiological effects of a general medical condition
- Nonpathological reactions to stress

Adapted from ref. [1].

TABLE 6.4. Talk therapy for adjustment disorders

- Counseling
- Crisis intervention
- Psychotherapy
- Group therapy
- Family therapy

Adapted from ref. [3].

TABLE 6.5. Goals of therapy for adjustment disorder

- Note significant dysfunction due to a stressor
- Help patients put their feelings into words (verbalization) rather than into destructive behaviors
- Assist the patient with better adaptation and mastery of stressors
- Clarify and interpret a stressor's meaning to a patient (e.g., address negative thinking, "catastrophizing")

Adapted from ref. [3].

TABLE 6.6. Examples of medications for sleep disturbance in adjustment disorder

- Diphenhydramine (Benadryl), hydroxyzine (Vistaril, Atarax)
- Trazodone (Desyrel)
- Zolpidem (Ambien, Ambien CR), zaleplon (Sonata), eszopiclone (Lunesta), ramelteon (Rozerem)
- Lorazepam (Ativan), clonazepam (Klonopin), temazepam (Restoril)

Adapted from ref. [2].

or removed, and establishing a support system (Table 6.5) [3]. The ultimate goal of intervention for the symptoms of an adjustment disorder is to improve patient functioning as quickly as possible. Psychotherapy and education help patients to recognize that the feelings of distress associated with an adjustment disorder are natural and expected, and the syndrome tends to be self-limited in many occasions [2].

Anxiety and tension associated with everyday life stressors usually do not require medication treatment. Some patients, however, experience symptoms such as sleep disturbance, overwhelming anxiety, and dysphoria, which may require medication in addition to talk therapy and education.

Short-term medication use can be helpful for patients who have a sleep disturbance associated with an adjustment disorder. These include antihistamines, sedative-hypnotics, and benzodiazepines (Table 6.6) [2]. Benzodiazepines such as alprazolam (Xanax), clonazepam (Klonopin), and lorazepam (Ativan) may also be helpful for daytime use for significant anxiety associated with severe life stresses.

Tricyclic antidepressants and buspirone (BuSpar) have been recommended instead of benzodiazepines for patients with a current or past history for alcohol abuse [3]. Several studies found that trazodone (Desyrel) was more effective than clorazepate (Tranxene) in the relief of anxious and depressed symptoms in patients with cancer and in HIV-positive patients [3]. Selective serotonin reuptake inhibitors (SSRIs) and serotonin-norepinephrine reuptake inhibitors (SNRIs) may help relieve dysphoric moods with minimal adverse effects and interactions [3].

The primary care practitioner must be vigilant and recognize that a patient may appear at a subthreshold level with a diagnosis of an adjustment disorder. This may indicate an early phase of a major mental disorder. If the patient's condition continues to evolve and worsen, the clinician must review the symptoms, perhaps revise the diagnosis, and appropriately treat the newly diagnosed mental disorder.

SUMMARY

An adjustment disorder is a subthreshold condition that can have several clinical features including anxiety. Stress has been determined as the cause for an adjustment disorder, and it can have an acute and chronic form. Adjustment disorders can comorbidly occur with other DSM-IV-TR diagnoses as well as be an initial phase for a developing major mental disorder. The practitioner must recognize that subthreshold syndromes such as adjustment disorder can themselves have significant psychopathology, and the disorder must be recognized and treated. Treatment is primarily psychotherapy, but medications may often be helpful and necessary. Adjustment disorder symptoms are often self-limited, and the general long-term outcome for adults appears to be good.

References

1. American Psychiatric Association. Diagnostic and Statistical Manual of Mental Disorders, 4th ed., text revision. Washington, DC: American Psychiatric Association, 2000.
2. Garlow SJ, Purselle D, D'Orio B. Psychiatric emergencies. In: Schatzberg AF, Nemeroff CB, eds. Textbook of Psychopharmacology, 3rd ed. Arlington, VA: American Psychiatric Publishing, 2004:1067–1082.
3. Strain JJ, Newcorn J. Adjustment disorders. In: Hales RE, Yudofsky SC, eds. Textbook of Clinical Psychiatry, 4th ed. Washington, DC: American Psychiatric Publishing, 2003:765–780.

7
Panic Disorder

James D. Helsley

Practitioners frequently encounter patients suffering from panic disorder symptoms. The symptoms may present in an obvious fashion or remain more subtle and hard to distinguish from common medical problems. The practitioner should always remain alert for the presentation of a patient with symptoms of panic disorder. The successful diagnosis and treatment of these patients is a deeply rewarding endeavor.

DEFINITION

According to the *Diagnostic and Statistical Manual of Mental Disorders*, 4th edition, text revision (DSM-IV-TR), panic disorder is defined as recurrent, unexpected panic attacks, which are episodes of intense fear and apprehension. The signs and symptoms of a panic attack include the following as listed in Table 7.1.

Panic attack symptom onset is rather abrupt and may occur without warning. Episodes may occur outside the home environment leading to agoraphobia [1]. The episode may be falsely interpreted as a heart attack, seizure, or stroke. There may be a sense of being "paralyzed" and unable to move. Often, a visit to the emergency room is the result. Patients may hyperventilate to the point of fainting, only to resume consciousness on the way to the hospital. The typical panic attack develops in intensity over approximately 10 minutes. Attacks may be full or partial in severity and occur unexpectedly, "out of the blue." This feature leads to anticipatory anxiety and avoidance of activities that might be associated with the attack [2]. Furthermore, life for the patient becomes disrupted and less satisfactory. The ramifications are quite considerable.

INCIDENCE AND PREVALENCE

Panic disorder is estimated to occur in 3.5% of the United States population. Females outnumber males by approximately 2:1. In the primary care setting, this disorder may exist in as many as

TABLE 7.1. Signs and symptoms of panic attack

- Overwhelming feeling of doom, fear of dying
- Palpitations, pounding heart, increased heart rate
- Sweating
- Sensation of shortness of breath or smothering
- Sensation of choking or blocked airway
- Feeling dizzy, light-headed, faint, or "fading away"
- Chills or hot flashes
- Fear of losing control or "going crazy"
- Chest pain, discomfort, pressure
- Feelings of unreality or being detached from oneself
- Numbness or tingling of hands, feet, lips
- Nausea, abdominal distress
- Shaking, trembling

Adapted from *Diagnostic and Statistical Manual of Mental Disorders,* 4th edition, text revision (DSM-IV-TR).

1 out of 10 patients [3] and may go unrecognized for long periods. The average age at onset of panic disorder is 20 to 30 years [3]. Approximately one third of patients recover with or without treatment and the remainder tends to relapse. Panic disorder patients utilize medical services considerably more than do non-panic patients. The perceived need by patients to seek medical attention for their symptoms leads to greater utilization of health care services. Anxiety disorders in general have been estimated to cost billions of dollars per year, including the cost of care, the utilization of services, and the loss of work productivity [1]. Many patients seek multiple evaluations by various specialists. Some patients transfer their care from practitioner to practitioner.

When patients present with symptoms of panic disorder, they are often desperate. This disorder can be disabling and can shake their confidence. They look to the practitioner for help and empathy, but may not be able to express their symptoms openly. Embarrassment and a fear that the practitioner will think they are "crazy" may interfere with the open dialogue necessary to proceed with diagnosis and treatment. Some cultures do not recognize mental health issues or allow patients to speak to the practitioner about these issues. Thus, recognizing and addressing the problem are major hurdles to overcome for the primary care practitioner. There is an understandable apprehension among many practitioners that mental health issues, including panic disorder in particular, will take much more time than they can afford to allot for one patient. Usually, it is simply the recognition and validation of the patient's concerns and apprehension that constitutes the practitioner's first duty. Once this is accomplished, the way is paved for pursuing a good treatment outcome.

FURTHER HISTORY: IMPORTANT AREAS TO CONSIDER DURING THE WORKUP

Since there are no specific tests or scans to confirm or deny a diagnosis of panic disorder, the practitioner must rely on an accurate and complete history in order to develop a clinical impression. Table 7.2 lists the important parts of the history to consider in patients suspected of having a panic disorder.

DIAGNOSIS

The diagnosis is established clinically by the history and the symptoms [4]. The clinician may proceed with treatment at this point. Some patients with anxiety disorders feel the need for multiple medical tests and investigations. The "ruling out" process is acceptable and sometimes can be therapeutic. The primary care practitioner should be honest and open with the patient when ordering tests such as the Holter monitor, lab tests for thyroid-stimulating hormone (TSH) and glucose, echocardiogram, electroencephalogram (EEG), and computed tomography (CT) scan of the head. It is wise to prepare the patient for a workup in which all results are negative. By doing so, the expectations of the patient are focused toward the ultimate goal of acceptance of

TABLE 7.2. History taking in panic disorder

- Onset of symptoms: When did the symptoms start? Was there a triggering event? Have there been any new medications? Do symptoms occur at night?
- Major life stressors, e.g., personal financial problems, relationship problems, job issues, family problems, school problems, loss of a loved one
- Previous diagnosis or treatment of an anxiety disorder or other psychiatric disorder
- Response (good or bad) to anxiolytic or other medication used in the past
- Use of alcohol, over-the-counter medications, illicit drugs, caffeine
- Is the patient depressed?
- Any psychotic symptoms such as hallucinations or paranoia
- Family history of mental health problems or general medical diseases
- Medical history and review of symptoms
- Could this diagnosis lead to a secondary gain?

Adapted from ref. [4].

the suspected primary diagnosis of panic disorder and acceptance of treatment recommendations. It is also a good idea to convey to patients early on that, despite their feeling that "everyday is my last on earth" or that they are going "crazy," these are symptoms of the disorder and not a likely reality. It is the extremely anxious mood that is the problem, and this anxiety is driving the patient's fears and concerns. Making this distinction and fully explaining the disorder to the patient is of paramount importance.

AGORAPHOBIA

Agora is the ancient Greek word for marketplace. Usually near the center of a city, it represented the gathering place for people and commerce. Thus, *agoraphobia* is defined as a fear of leaving home or being in situations that involve crowds where easy escape may be difficult, such as malls, airplanes, restaurants, theaters, stadiums, and arenas. The patient who suffers from agoraphobia may develop panic attacks when exposed to these types of situations. In turn, patients will "wall off" their life and even become homebound. Numerous excuses are often developed by the patient to avoid being in situations that might compound the agoraphobia/panic complex. This behavior can be especially disabling for the patient and a cause for distress among family members. Panic disorder may exist with or without agoraphobia [4].

ETIOLOGY THEORIES

The exact cause of panic disorder is not known. There have a number of theories that have been proposed [1]:

- Catastrophic misinterpretation: This concept is based on the premise that sensory input is not identified by the brain as attributable to a specific cause. This error in identification allows for a misinterpretation of catastrophic proportions leading to considerable autonomic discharge.
- Anxiety sensitivity: The theory in this instance is that patients are hypersensitive to environmental stimuli. There is no misinterpretation of sensory input, but more a magnification of known and understood sensations.
- Panic conditioning: Upon experiencing the first panic attack, the patient may develop neural pathways that are "fast-track" routes for successive stimuli in the future. In this way, the panic attack occurs more easily.
- Separation: This concept stems from the belief that separation anxiety early in life leads to the panic attack complex later in young adulthood. Subsequent circumstances that center on

separation (e.g., divorce) lead to panic attacks as the anxiety response.

- False suffocation: In this theoretical construct, the patient is thought to have a dysregulation of the otherwise normal response to suffocation. If CO_2 or lactate levels rise even modestly, the brain may interpret it as suffocation and produce the panic response.

NEUROBIOLOGY

Neuroimaging studies using functional magnetic resonance imaging (fMRI), positive emission tomography (PET), and other modalities have shown changes in functional anatomy in patients with panic disorder [1,2]. There is a considerable amount of evidence supporting the premise of neurotransmitter dysregulation, both excess and deficiency, in these patients [1]:

- Serotonin: It is thought that serotonin activity is necessary for the action of conditioning pathways. Given a relative lack of serotonin in the suppressive feedback loops, the patient may not be able to inhibit the response to sensory stimuli. The patient then becomes overwhelmed with somatic sensory input and essentially decompensates and has a panic attack.
- Norepinephrine: Distributed throughout the autonomic nervous system are norepinephrine receptors that produce the physiologic effects of stimulation or arousal. It has been postulated that panic disorder patients possess a heightened activity or sensitivity to norepinephrine.

Whatever the origins of panic disorder, suffice it to say that it is a complex disease with multiple cognitive and neurobiological causes. Future research may provide answers that elude us currently.

TREATMENT

The initial step in the treatment of panic disorder is patient education [5]. Helping patients understand what panic disorder represents to them individually is a useful technique. It is important to validate that their sensations and symptoms are real. They certainly are! A very useful technique is to convey to the patient in a calming tone that the diagnosis is real, that panic is a relatively common condition, and very treatable. The practitioner should keep expectations and treatment discussions on a reasonable and practical level. A realistic approach is to stress that there are no miracle cures, but treatment helps people lead normal lives.

Lifestyle changes may be very helpful. Reducing excessive intake of caffeine may help (greater than three beverages per day is excessive). Even small amounts of caffeine can be anxiogenic. Decaffeinated beverages may contain a small amount of caffeine, enough to affect susceptible patients. Exogenous adrenergic stimulants (e.g., decongestants and certain herbal and over-the-counter substances) should be limited. Elimination and modification of any known triggers, if feasible, can be helpful. An exercise program has been shown to reduce panic episodes [6].

MEDICATION

Several classes of medications have been demonstrated to be effective in the treatment of panic disorder. The two major classes are the benzodiazepines and the selective serotonin reuptake inhibitors (SSRIs). The serotonin-norepinephrine reuptake inhibitor (SNRI) venlafaxine (Effexor XR) is effective in treating panic disorder as well.

Benzodiazepines

Rapid-onset, short-acting tranquilizers help by aborting or limiting panic episodes [7]. Alprazolam (Xanax) and lorazepam (Ativan) are commonly used. Clonazepam (Klonopin) is long acting and may work more efficiently in some patients [7]. Table 7.3 lists three commonly used benzodiazepines for panic disorder. These medications have been approved by the Food and Drug Administration (FDA) for use in panic disorder patients.

Selective Serotonin Reuptake Inhibitors

The SSRIs are invaluable in the long-term treatment and prevention of panic episodes [1,2,4,8–10]. These medications work well,

TABLE 7.3. Benzodiazepines

Drug name	Dosage supplied	Onset	Half-life	Starting dosage
Alprazolam (Xanax)	0.25 mg 0.5 mg 1 mg	15–30 minutes	12 hours	0.25–0.5 mg b.i.d.
Lorazepam (Ativan)	0.5 mg 1 mg 2 mg	15–30 minutes	14 hours	0.5 mg b.i.d.
Clonazepam (Klonopin)	0.5 mg 1 mg 2 mg	30–60 minutes	25 hours	0.5 mg b.i.d.

Adapted from ref. [7].

TABLE 7.4. Selective serotonin reuptake inhibitors (FDA approved)

Drug name	Dosage supplied	Maximum dosage/day	Half-life	Starting dosage
Sertraline (Zoloft)	25 mg 50 mg 100 mg	200 mg	25 hours	25 mg q.d.
Paroxetine (Paxil, Paxil CR)	Paxil: 10 mg 20 mg 30 mg 40 mg	Paxil: 60 mg	21 hours	10 mg q.d.
	CR: 12.5 mg 25 mg 37.5 mg	CR: 75 mg	CR: 21 hours	CR: 12.5 mg q.d.
Fluoxetine (Prozac)	10 mg 20 mg 40 mg	80 mg	4–6 days	10 mg q.d.

Adapted from ref. [2].

are generally well tolerated, and regarded as safe in most cases [10]. This class of medications is regarded as the primary treatment for most patients. While the benzodiazepines work nicely to control panic symptoms, the SSRIs may help to prevent panic attacks altogether. Table 7.4 lists several SSRI medications that have been FDA approved for indications of panic disorder.

Other Medication Treatments
Table 7.5 lists other medications that may be effective for panic disorder. Venlafaxine (Effexor XR) is approved for use by the FDA for the treatment of panic disorder. Fluvoxamine (Luvox), citalopram (Celexa), and escitalopram (Lexapro) are not specifically approved by the FDA for the treatment of panic disorder, but may be useful therapies in some patients.

FURTHER DRUG CONSIDERATIONS
The following medications are not FDA approved but may have usefulness as single agent therapy or in combination with an SSRI for panic disorder:

• Bupropion (Wellbutrin XL): This is not an SSRI. It works by inhibiting dopamine and norepinephrine reuptake. It may have some degree of effect on panic disorder, especially when associated with depression [10]. It can make panic worse as well. When

TABLE 7.5. Other drugs useful in treatment of panic disorder

Drug name	Dosage supplied	Maximum dosage/day	Half-life	Starting dosage
Venlafaxine (Effexor XR) FDA approved	37.5 mg 75 mg 150 mg	225 mg	11 hours	37.5 mg q.d.
Fluvoxamine (Luvox)	25 mg 50 mg 100 mg	300 mg	15 hours	25 mg q.d.
Citalopram (Celexa)	10 mg 20 mg 40 mg	60 mg	35 hours	10 mg q.d.
Escitalopram (Lexapro)	5 mg 10 mg 20 mg	40 mg	30 hours	5 mg q.d.

Adapted from ref. [2].

used in panic disorder, lower doses (150 mg per day to start) are recommended.

- Buspirone (BuSpar): This medication may be helpful in treating generalized anxiety disorder symptoms; however, for panic disorder it is not much better than a placebo [4]. This drug really has no use as a stand-alone medication in panic disorder.
- Atypical antipsychotics: Some early studies have shown olanzapine (Zyprexa) as effective for panic disorder. Evidence is shallow, however. Augmentation of SSRI therapy with the newer atypical antipsychotics may show some promise. Aripiprazole (Abilify) or ziprasidone (Geodon) may make a nice "add-on" treatment to baseline SSRI therapy. Further investigation is necessary.
- Tricyclic antidepressants (TCAs): The TCAs were the mainstay of medical therapy for years. Clomipramine (Anafranil), amitriptyline (Elavil), nortriptyline (Pamelor), imipramine (Tofranil), desipramine (Norpramin), and doxepin (Sinequan) have been used for years but are increasingly a thing of the past. Side effects of sedation, dry mouth, potential cardiac dysrhythmia, and urinary retention, as well as the effectiveness and safety of SSRIs, have led to the decline in tricyclic use. TCAs are options if other treatments fail.
- Duloxetine (Cymbalta): There are no published studies demonstrating the use of duloxetine in patients with panic disorder. To this point, the literature demonstrates only a case report [11]. Its use in the future for panic disorder and other anxiety disorders may show promise.

GENERAL CONSIDERATIONS OF TREATMENT

Benzodiazepine Abuse Potential

Selective serotonin reuptake inhibitor and benzodiazepine therapy are first-line therapy in panic disorder [4,5]. As with many other treatments, it is important to start with a low dose and advance it as tolerated. It is best to titrate doses of medication upward cautiously while attempting to reach a balance among [1] control of symptoms, [2] intolerance, and [3] side effects.

The benzodiazepines work to control symptoms quickly, usually within 15 to 30 minutes. In many cases, benzodiazepines provide comfort to the patient in just knowing that immediate or abortive relief is nearby. They are extremely helpful medications for the patient who suffers from panic disorder and should not be summarily dismissed by the practitioner out of a fear of prescribing a controlled substance. Careless prescribing by a practitioner is obviously unwise, yet not offering a safe, useful, and effective medication to a patient in need could be construed as just as unwise. Although abuse and dependence are potential concerns with benzodiazepines [12], this problem is usually avoidable by doing the following:

1. Using only the dose necessary to control symptoms
2. Using only when needed for panic attacks even if this requires regular use for a period of time
3. Monitoring patients closely and reviewing use at each visit
4. Keeping good records to track usage and refills

Selective serotonin reuptake inhibitor therapy at its optimum will generally prevent panic attacks altogether. At that point, benzodiazepines are helpful for breakthrough or rescue treatment.

Comorbidity

The primary care practitioner must always be alert for comorbidity. Coexistent depression and other mood disorders, alcohol and other substance abuse (many patients prefer to self-medicate), and other anxiety disorders may lurk in the shadows behind panic disorder symptoms [1,2]. Many patients rely on alcohol or other drugs, for example, marijuana or narcotics, to control the symptoms of panic disorder [5,7,13]. Self-medication is a common and serious problem. Since panic disorder is coupled with a fear of losing control, patients may find it more acceptable to treat themselves than to visit a practitioner for an appropriate diagnosis and treatment. During therapy, if the patient is not responding to medication treatment as expected, the practitioner must consider other diagnoses [2].

Treatment Compliance

As with many illnesses, the lack of compliance with medication can be a serious problem. Periodic reexamination and evaluation, ongoing review of medication, solicitation for side effects, and open discussion about price and affordability will help address compliance issues preemptively. Panic disorder may exist for years and treatment may need to be continued for years to improve the patient's quality of life.

COGNITIVE BEHAVIOR THERAPY

Primary care physicians and mid-level providers are in a unique position to provide emotional support for panic disorder [4]. Simply listening to the patient in a calm and empathetic manner is extremely crucial to a successful outcome. When time constraints are a problem, a referral may be made to a therapist who can listen, and provide nonjudgmental opinions and recommendations in a supportive atmosphere.

One overriding concern of patients who suffer from panic disorder is apprehension and doom and that collapse of their world is imminent. This can be a very disabling state for the patient. Reassurance and validation by the practitioner can help patients to become better educated about the problem. This leads to a decrease in their fear and an increase in their motivation and involvement. This can only help to improve the outcome.

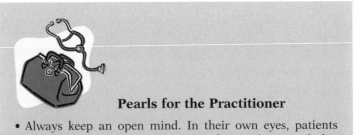

Pearls for the Practitioner

- Always keep an open mind. In their own eyes, patients with panic disorder are in a state of crisis that is real, distressing, and threatening to their well-being.
- Not all that looks like panic is panic. Some medical diseases can produce symptoms similar to those seen in panic disorder. These diseases may include hyperthyroidism, chronic obstructive pulmonary disease, coronary heart disease, seizure disorder, stroke, Meniere's syndrome, anemia, and others.

- The calming approach by the practitioner is crucial. If the patient who feels out of control is allowed to witness the practitioner "in control," the way is opened for a successful outcome.
- Use a lead-in question to address panic and anxiety symptoms that is not judgmental. Some patients are reluctant to discuss the symptoms of panic disorder. Open-ended questions usually work the best to give the patient an opportunity to provide the practitioner with a more detailed history. For example, "How are your nerves doing lately?" and "Are you sleeping OK? are useful questions to expand the history.
- Become familiar with several medications and center your treatment around those drugs. It is not necessary to know all drugs and drug classes to treat panic disorder patients. Keeping a few in mind will allow the practitioner to have a working comfort level with those medications. Often the practitioner's personal first-line treatment regimen is effective and all that is needed to make for successful treatment. Since every patient may not respond to a certain medication exactly the same way, a subsequent follow-up visit will allow the practitioner time to adjust or change the medication.
- The practitioner does not have to do the entire workup, intervention, cognitive behavior therapy, and drug therapy in one visit. Primary care practitioners are busy people. Breaking up the intervention, workup, and treatment into several visits will allow the busy practitioner to handle the panic disorder patient properly and efficiently without causing a scheduling catastrophe in the office.
- Referral to another provider, such as a psychiatrist, might be necessary. Many panic disorder patients can be treated quite well by the primary care practitioner. Many practitioners are quite capable of treating panic disorder with excellent outcome. If treatment of the patient diagnosed with panic disorder is not proceeding according to expectations, then consider referral.
- Comorbidity is common. Sometimes a patient will suffer from panic disorder as the sole diagnosis. In many instances, the patient may also suffer from major depression, obsessive-compulsive disorder, social anxiety disorder, posttraumatic stress disorder, bipolar disorder, or other psychiatric diagnoses. It is best to keep an open mind when treating panic disorder and remain alert for the presence of other psychiatric illness.

Continued

Continued

- Personality disorders can occur simultaneously with panic disorder. Many patients with panic disorder are living a distressed life any truly desire help from the practitioner. Patients who are manipulative, histrionic, or seeking secondary gain may also have panic disorder. These patients require more time and effort from the practitioner to sort out the issues in their care. These patients usually are more demanding and difficult.
- Patients change over time. As with most other health care issues, patients with panic disorder change with time. Some have improvement of symptoms and some become worse. Periodic reassessment by the practitioner is crucial to good long-term care.

SUMMARY

Panic disorder is a common, potentially disabling problem commonly seen in primary care. The presentation may not always be obvious. Many social and cultural issues preclude a prompt diagnosis [14]. Upon evaluation and treatment, the patient can receive support, medication, and cognitive therapy. The successful recognition and treatment of panic disorders can be one of the most gratifying experiences in the practice of medicine.

References

1. Pollack M, et al. Panic disorder: broadening conceptualizations and improving treatment. CNS Spectrums Academic Suppl 2005;10(9, suppl 12):4–39.
2. Bystritsky A, Williams K. Panic disorder. In: Rakel R, Bope E, eds. Conn's Current Therapy. Philadelphia: Saunders, 2006:1374–1379.
3. Vanin J, Vanin S. Blocking the cycle of panic disorder. Postgrad Med 1999;105(5):141–148.
4. Roy-Byrne P, Wagner A, Schraufnagel T. Understanding and treating panic disorder in the primary care setting. J Clin Psychiatry 2005;66(suppl 4):16–22
5. Abelson J, Liberzon I, Young E, Khan S. Cognitive modulation of the endocrine stress response to the pharmacologic challenge in normal and panic disorder subjects. Arch Gen Psychiatry 2005;62:668–675.
6. Strohle A, Feller C, Onken M, Godermann F, Heinz A, Dimeo F. The acute anti-panic activity of aerobic exercise. Am J Psychiatry 2005;162(12):2376–2378.
7. Shearer S, Gordon L. The patient with excessive worry. Am Fam Physician March 15 2006;73(6):1049–1056.

8. Hollander E, Simeon D. Anxiety disorders. In: Hales R, Yudofsky S, eds. Textbook of Clinical Psychiatry, 4th ed. Washington, DC: American Psychiatric Publishing, 2003:543–565.

9. Panic disorder. In: Chan P, Thomas D, McKinley E, Stanford E, eds. Outpatient and Primary Care Medicine. Laguna Hills, CA: Current Clinical Strategies Publishing, 2005:240–243.

10. Pollack M. The pharmacotherapy of panic disorder. J Clin Psychiatry 2005;66(suppl 4):23–27.

11. Crippa J, Zuardi A. Duloxetine in the treatment of panic disorder. Int J Neuropsychopharmacol 2005;November 17:1–2.

12. Gale C, Oakley-Browne M. Generalised anxiety disorder. IN: Tovey D, ed. Clinical Concise Evidence, vol. 14. London: BMJ Publishing Group, 2005:334–336.

13. Ninan P, Dunlop B. Neurobiology and etiology of panic disorder. J Clin Psychiatry 2005;66(suppl 4):3–7.

14. Simon N, Fischmann D. The implications of medical and psychiatric co-morbidity with panic disorder. J Clin Psychiatry 2005;66(suppl 4):8–15.

8
Specific Phobia

John R. Vanin

Specific phobia, formerly called simple phobia, is an anxiety disorder characterized by a marked and persistent fear of specific objects, situations, or activities [1–3]. Patients know their fear is excessive or unreasonable but are unable to overcome it. The possibility of encountering a phobic stimulus causes anticipatory anxiety. The individual either avoids or endures the object or situation with dread [2]. Ultimately this may lead to great distress or impairment in functioning and to a disorder [4]. Tables 8.1 and 8.2 list the diagnostic criteria for specific phobia [1] and the different subtypes [1,2].

The specific phobia subtypes are distinct, and they differ regarding age and mode of onset, physiological responses, and family aggregation [2]. The focus of the fear in specific phobia may vary (Table 8.3) [1]. The blood-injection-injury subtype for example is often associated with a strong vasovagal response, and many patients faint [1]. This type of phobia may lead to academic and occupational distress, and to medical problems because a person may avoid medical or dental care. A 2001 survey on dental practice stress found that dealing with patient anxiety was a major cause of stress among dentists and that the most common patient fears included fear of injections and a sense of not being in control [5]. The fear of choking may cause patients to be noncompliant with taking their medications because of swallowing concerns with tablets or capsules.

The ranking of the frequency of social phobia subtypes appearing in clinical settings is as follows: situational, natural environment, blood-injection-injury, and animals [1]. Patients may have more than one subtype of specific phobia and the likelihood of having another phobia within a subtype increases if a patient has one phobia of a specific subtype [1].

Many specific phobias begin in childhood and may spontaneously disappear. Some patients develop phobias in late adolescence or early adulthood, which are less likely to spontaneously

TABLE 8.1. Diagnostic criteria for specific phobia

- Excessive or unreasonable fear that is marked and persistent
- Fear is cued by the anticipation of or the presence of the specific object or situation
- An immediate anxiety response usually occurs with exposure to the phobic stimulus; the anxiety may take the form of a panic attack
- Recognition that the fear is excessive and unreasonable
- Phobic situation is avoided or endured with intense anxiety or distress
- Significant interference by the avoidance, anxious anticipation, or distress of the feared situation with the individual's normal routine, occupational or academic functioning, social activities, relationships, or considerable distress about having the phobia
- At least 6 months duration in individuals younger than 18 years
- Another mental disorder does not better account for the anxiety, panic attacks, or phobic avoidance of the specific object or situation

Adapted from ref. [1].

TABLE 8.2. Subtypes of specific phobia

Subtype	Examples
Animal	Snakes, dogs, mice, insects, spiders
Natural environment	Storms, thunder, lightening, water, wind, heights
Situational	Tunnels, bridges, elevators, flying, cars, closed spaces
Blood-injection-injury	Receiving an injection, invasive medical procedures, seeing blood or an injury
Other	Choking, vomiting, contracting an illness

Adapted from refs. [1] and [2].

TABLE 8.3. Focus of fear in specific phobia

- Anticipated harm from object or situation
- Concerns about losing control
- Concerns about panicking
- Somatic symptoms (e.g., shortness of breath, increased heart rate)
- Fainting

Adapted from ref. [1].

disappear [6]. The fear in specific phobias usually concerns some dire outcome that the patient believes may result from contact with the object or situation rather than the object or situation itself. Reassurance does not reduce the patient's fear despite their acknowledgment that there is really nothing to fear. When not in the feared situation, the person may admit that the fear is unreasonable and joke about the feared object or situation.

ASSOCIATED FEATURES

Specific phobias may significantly interfere with a person's life including their job, school, or social activities. For example, the fear of the sight of blood can be a disabling condition for a health care practitioner. Also, a sales representative with a flying phobia may lose a job promotion if frequent flying is required.

It is important for the primary care practitioner to note that other disorders may resemble specific phobias. For example, an individual with social anxiety may get very apprehensive or panicky regarding a medical appointment because of the general fear of the social interaction, whereas an individual with specific phobia might fear a particular procedure such as blood drawing or an injection. Another example is an individual with panic disorder who may avoid flying or driving because of the fear of having a panic attack in the plane or car, whereas an individual with specific phobia may fear a plane crash or an automobile accident.

Specific phobias often coexist with other psychiatric disorders such as a mood disorder, substance use disorder, and other anxiety disorders [1]. The rates of comorbidity in community settings range from 50% to 80%, but in clinical settings, specific phobias are rarely the focus of clinical attention because they are usually associated with less distress or functional problems than the comorbid diagnosis [1].

EPIDEMIOLOGY

Specific phobias are common in the general population but individuals rarely warrant a diagnosis or seek treatment because of insufficient distress or impairment [2]. According to the National Comorbidity Survey Replication, the 12-month prevalence of specific phobia is 8.7% and the lifetime prevalence is 12.5% [7,8]. Prevalence rates vary for the specific phobia subtypes and decline for the elderly [1]. Women are affected more than twice as often as men [2]. Age at onset is often before the age of 7 years for the common specific phobias such as insect, blood, darkness, animal, and injury [4]. The content of the phobias varies with the ethnicity and culture [3]. Specific phobias may have strong family patterns [1].

ONSET

The symptoms of a specific phobia usually first occur in children or early adolescence and may occur at a younger age for women versus men [1]. Ages at onset for the various subtypes of specific

TABLE 8.4. Age at onset for specific phobia subtypes

Subtype	Age of onset
Situational	Childhood; mid-20s
Natural environment	Childhood; early adulthood
Animal	Childhood
Blood-injection-injury	Childhood

Adapted from ref. [1].

TABLE 8.5. Predisposing factors to specific phobia onset

- Traumatic events
- Unexpected panic attacks
- Observation of others undergoing trauma
- Observation of others demonstrating fearfulness
- Informational transmission (e.g., parental danger warnings, media coverage of disasters/crashes)

Adapted from ref. [1].

phobia are listed in Table 8.4 [1]. Predisposing factors to the onset of specific phobias are listed in Table 8.5 [1].

ETIOLOGY

There are many theories regarding the formation of phobic symptoms (Table 8.6) [2,3]. These include psychodynamic, behavioral, and biological theories. Freud initially developed a psychological theory of phobic symptom formation and later reconceptualized this theory into his structural theory [2]. The psychodynamic approach focuses on symbolic meanings of the phobic object and conflicts, which the phobia serves to avoid [2].

In behavioral theory, phobic anxiety is thought to be a conditioned response (learning theory) acquired through association of the phobic object (conditioned stimulus) with a noxious experience (unconditioned stimulus) [2]. Avoidance of the phobic object reduces or prevents conditioned anxiety. Behavioral techniques (deconditioning) are relatively successful in the treatment of specific phobias.

Hollander and Simeon noted Fyer's description of various etiology models of specific phobias. One is based on a modified conditioning model, which involves four points (Table 8.7) [2]. Another describes the nonassociative model, which proposes that each species has

TABLE 8.6. Theories of phobic symptom formation

- Psychodynamic
- Behavioral
- Biological
- Environmental

Adapted from refs. [2] and [3].

TABLE 8.7. Modified conditioning model for specific phobia

- An initial aversive event is not recalled by many phobic patients. This suggests if such an event had occurred, an amygdala-based emotional memory must have encoded the memory (not by hippocampus-based episodic memory). This process either occurred before age 3 years or was encoded under conditions that were highly stressful.
- Most human phobias involve a small number of objects. There may be an evolutionary-based biological preparedness for specific stimuli that would be conditioned easily but extinguished with difficulty.
- Genetic vulnerabilities or previous experiences may play a role in specific phobia because developing a phobic reaction after exposure to a certain stimulus occurs only in a minority of individuals.
- Despite belief and evidence that there is nothing to fear, in the absence of specific interventions, most phobias are extinction resistant.

Adapted from ref. [2].

certain fears that are innate and a part of normal development [2]. In specific phobia, there may be a failure to habituate over time to these fears because of factors such as individual vulnerability, life stressors, or unsafe environments [2].

Specific phobias have a high familial transmission [2]. Hollander and Simeon cited a large study of phobias in twins by Kender et al., that found depending on the particular phobia, genetic factors mostly accounted for the familial aggregation [2]. There is increasing data in the genetics of fear conditioning and extinction regarding variations in neuroendocrine receptors, monoamine receptors, and amino acid receptors [3]. Environmental factors also play a significant role in phobic avoidance including fear conditioning [3].

Brain imaging studies of specific phobia have been inconclusive, but functional imaging in humans shows that the amygdala is activated by the presentation of masked fearful expressions [2,3]. The amygdala plays a key role in the psychobiology of fear conditioning and extinction [3]. The neurocircuits of the amygdala involve a range of different neurotransmitters including serotonin, norepinephrine, glutamate, and γ-aminobenzoic acid (GABA).

From an evolutionary perspective, the mechanisms of specific phobia may serve a survival purpose to detect and avoid harmful stimuli. Mammals have a complex emotional learning and functional alarm system that may sometimes be triggered too little or too often [3].

TREATMENT

Treatment of specific phobias includes cognitive-behavioral therapy, particularly exposure (Table 8.8) [9]. Pharmacotherapy may also be helpful for some patients. Medications such as anxiolytics (e.g., benzodiazepines) or β-adrenergic receptor antagonists may be helpful to assist the patient in the early stages of exposure therapy [6]. If panic attacks are part of the phobic symptomatology, antipanic medication may be indicated [2].

Therapy

Cognitive-behavioral strategies often combine relaxation techniques (e.g., deep breathing exercises, muscle relaxation), a systematic or graded exposure to the avoided object or situation, and psychoeducation [6]. The practitioner can discuss information about the disorder and the treatment in an interactive manner so that the patient is more likely to understand the concepts and implement the therapy. Graded exposure consists of either progressively imagining the feared situation (imaginal exposure) or actually being directly exposed to feared stimuli (in vivo exposure) [2,4]. The patient begins with the least stressful mild fears

TABLE 8.8. Cognitive and behavioral therapies

- Emphasize psychoeducation
- Typically use homework and self-help assignments
- Psychiatric illness is objectively assessed and is an integral part of treatment
- Therapeutic methods are generally structured, directive, and require activity by the therapist
- Time-limited therapies
- Empirical evidence validates and guides therapeutic technique choices

Adapted from ref. [9].

and gradually progresses to more significant fears [4]. Imagery techniques may precede actual exposure to the feared stimuli. Ungraded exposure (flooding) can occur in both imaginal and actual exposure and consists of patients initially confronting the most stressful fears. Exposure techniques can be used in individual as well as group settings.

The primary care practitioner can help patients deal with a phobic stimulus by first describing an image and allowing the patients to use their imagination. The clinician can help patients confront the feared thoughts, images, and memories and better understand and face their fears. Subsequently, the patients can get involved in real contact with the object or situation until they are calmer and have a sense of mastery over the situation. Increasing exposure to the feared object or situation without aversive consequences allows patients to break the cycle of fearfulness that is reinforced by avoidance and escape behaviors [9]. Perhaps the brief use of a benzodiazepine can facilitate the exposure to the feared stimulus. Sometimes there is a challenge in convincing patients that exposure therapy will be beneficial.

Other efficacious treatments include participant modeling, contingency management, and cognitive exercises such as self-monitoring (keeping a diary of thoughts and behaviors), positive self-talk, and thought-stopping techniques [4]. No specific exposure technique has been shown to be superior to other techniques or is specifically indicated for particular subtypes of phobias [2].

Pharmacotherapy

Medications generally do not appear to be useful as a first-line treatment for specific phobia. Anxiolytics or β-adrenergic receptor blockers may be helpful at the initial stages of exposure therapy [6,10]. The benefits of exposure may also be extended by medication augmentation [11]. Benzodiazepines used intermittently may be helpful in the acute treatment of somatic anxiety [11]. Serotonergic medications are efficacious in treating fear and avoidance of various anxiety disorders. A small study showed 60% of the patients taking paroxetine for specific phobia responded versus 17% taking placebo [11]. Antipanic medication such as benzodiazepines and selective serotonin reuptake inhibitors may be indicated in patients who have panic attacks as part of their phobic symptomatology [2,10,12].

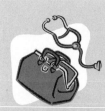

Pearls for the Practitioner

- Specific phobia is an anxiety disorder characterized by a marked and persistent fear of specific objects, situations, or activities.
- Specific phobia has several distinct subtypes, which may lead to great distress or impairment of functioning.
- Many childhood specific phobias disappear spontaneously, but some phobias that develop in adolescence or early adulthood are less likely to spontaneously disappear.
- Specific phobias affect over six million American adults and may coexist with other psychiatric disorders such as mood disorders, substance use disorders, and other anxiety disorders.
- Theories regarding the formation of phobic symptoms include psychodynamic, behavioral, biological, and environmental.
- Specific phobia development from an evolutionary perspective includes serving as a survival mechanism to detect and avoid harmful stimuli.
- Treatment of specific phobia includes cognitive behavior therapy as well as medication.

SUMMARY

The primary care practitioner must encourage patients with specific phobia to identify the phobic stimulus, confront the object or situation, experience the anxiety, and ultimately conquer their fears [10]. The process can be slow and time-consuming. Referral to a skilled therapist may be indicated. A persistent approach by the practitioner with a patient who constantly practices can yield positive results.

References

1. American Psychiatric Association. Diagnostic and Statistical Manual of Mental Disorders, 4th ed., text revision. Washington, DC: American Psychiatric Association, 2000.

2. Hollander E, Simeon D. Anxiety disorders. In: Hales RE, Yudofsky SC, eds. Textbook of Clinical Psychiatry, 4th ed. Washington, DC: American Psychiatric Publishing, 2003:543–630.

3. Stein DJ, Matsunaga H. Specific phobia: a disorder of fear conditioning and extinction. CNS Spectr 2006;11:248–251.

4. Bernstein GA, Layne AE. Separation anxiety disorder and other anxiety disorders. In: Sadock BJ, Sadock VA, eds. Sadock's Comprehensive Textbook of Psychiatry, 8th ed., vol. 2. Philadelphia: Lippincott Williams & Wilkins, 2005:3292–3302.

5. Dental Fears and Phobias. http:/dentistry.about.com/od/dentalfacts/a/fearsphobias.htm

6. Shader RI, Greenblatt DJ. Approaches to the treatment of anxiety states. In: Shader RI, ed. Manual of Psychiatric Therapeutics, 3rd ed. Philadelphia: Lippincott Williams & Wilkins, 2003:184–209.

7. Kessler RC, Chiu WT, Demler O, Walters EE. Prevalence, severity, and comorbidity of 12-month DSM-IV disorders in the national comorbidity survey replication. Arch Gen Psychiatry 2005;62:617–627.

8. Kessler RC, Berglund P, Demler O, Jin R, Walters EE. Lifetime prevalence and age-of-onset distributions of DSM-IV disorders in the national comorbidity survey replication. Arch Gen Psychiatry 2005;62:593–601.

9. Friedman ES, Thase ME, Wright JH. Cognitive and behavioral therapies. In: Tasman A, Kay J, Lieberman JA, eds. Psychiatry Therapeutics, 2nd ed. West Sussex: John Wiley & Sons, 2003:55–79.

10. Berman CW. Fall from perfection: a case of phobia. CNS News 2005(September), 7:43.

11. Davidson JRT, Connor KM. Treatment of anxiety disorders. In: Schatzberg AF, Nemeroff CB, eds. Textbook of Psychopharmacology, 3rd ed. Arlington, VA: American Psychiatric Publishing, 2004:913–934.

12. Berman CW. Facing our fears: effective treatment of phobias. CNS News 2001(April), 2:5.

9
Social Phobia
(Social Anxiety Disorder)

James D. Helsley

Social phobia is a common disorder with an approximate 13% lifetime prevalence [1]. Social phobia may also be referred to as social anxiety disorder (SAD). Onset of SAD is usually in adolescence or early adulthood and may be acute or insidious [1]. The acute onset follows a specific humiliating event that likely has occurred in childhood or early adolescence. Social anxiety disorder in its milder form may be a common event in many people.

Almost everyone has experienced apprehension when speaking in front of the class during one's early school years. For some, the fear, anxiety, and apprehension may persist, expand, and worsen into adulthood, resulting in avoidance behaviors and considerable disability. Social anxiety often creates a hindrance to success and happiness. Social anxiety, panic disorder, and posttraumatic stress disorder together may have more impact on quality of life and poorer levels of functioning than the combined effect of chronic medical illnesses and depression [2].

DEFINITION
The *Diagnostic and Statistical Manual of Mental Disorders*, 4th edition, text revision (DSM-IV-TR) defines social phobia (social anxiety disorder) as a marked and persistent fear of one or more social/performance situations. The exposure to the inciting situation causes the development of anxiety that may meet the criteria for a panic attack [3]. The fear and anticipatory anxiety of social anxiety disorder are excessive and often lead to avoidance behaviors. The level of distress is marked and may lead to the patient's inability to successfully function.

DIAGNOSIS
The diagnosis of SAD is made by taking an appropriate psychiatric history, which should include the patient's current symptoms, the time of symptom origin, inciting events, and efforts at resolution of the

anxiety. Social anxiety symptoms may originate in childhood or adolescence. The patient may be affected for many years before seeking help and treatment [4].

Common situations that may produce the symptoms of social anxiety disorder include the following [5]:

- Public speaking
- Public performance
- Using public restrooms
- Meeting someone new or someone "important"
- Attending social events (e.g., meetings, dances, family gatherings)
- Being observed during an activity
- Required participation in group activities

Comorbidity is very common in patients suffering from SAD. Half of these patients may suffer from coexistent depression, drug abuse, or alcohol abuse [5]. Whether the substance abuse is a preceding event to the SAD or vice versa is not clear. Screening for substance use and major depressive symptoms during the evaluation of a patient suspected of having social anxiety disorder is an important step.

There are three subtypes of social anxiety disorder: [1] generalized social anxiety disorder, [2] nongeneralized social anxiety disorder, and [3] performance/public-speaking phobia [6]. While making the distinction may have some implication in treatment, it is likely that the primary care practitioner will find it useful to make the diagnosis as the entire disorder alone and not strive to define a subtype.

Several published rating scales are helpful in making the diagnosis of SAD [7]:

1. Brief Fear of Negative Evaluation Scale (Brief-FNE), © Mark Leary
2. Fear Questionnaire (FQ), © Isaac Marks, M.D.
3. Liebowitz Social Anxiety Scale (LSAS), © Dr. Michael Liebowitz
4. Social Phobia and Anxiety Inventory (SPAI), © Samuel Turner, Ph.D., Deborah Beidel, Ph.D., Constance Dancu, Ph.D.

These scales usually take less than 20 minutes to administer and can be helpful in supporting the clinical diagnosis of SAD. The first two listed are self-administered by the patient, and the third and fourth are administered by a clinician or other trained individual.

AVOIDANT PERSONALITY DISORDER

The DSM-IV-TR describes an avoidant personality disorder as a pervasive pattern of behavior where the patient is preoccupied with [1] social inhibition, [2] an intense fear of negative evaluation by others, and [3] marked feelings of inadequacy [3]. While similar, there are differences between the symptoms of SAD and avoidant personality disorder. In general, patients with avoidant personality disorder are intensely concerned with criticism or rejection in social situations. There is an avoidance of social activities where the possibility of disapproval may occur. Feelings of inadequacy are persistent, and the patient has a marked fear of taking risks.

On the other hand, the diagnosis of SAD centers on the anxious experiences of worry, fear, and apprehension that may accompany exposure to the social situation where performance of some degree is required or expected. In addition, the patient understands that the fear is excessive and unreasonable.

TREATMENT

Psychotherapy

Treatment consists of two main avenues of approach. Cognitive behavior therapy (CBT), a form of psychotherapy, is considered by some to be the first-line treatment of choice for SAD [8]. It may be administered by the primary care practitioner in the office setting. Usually serial appointments are established that involve relaxation techniques and visualization of the phobia-inciting stimulus. The patient is guided through a period of progressive desensitization by the repeated exposure to the phobic situation. In this way, the anxiety behavior associated with the phobia is diminished or eliminated. Cognitive behavior therapy is discussed in detail in Chapter 5.

Some practitioners may not feel comfortable doing psychotherapy. Referral to an experienced therapist may be necessary for some patients.

Pharmacological Treatment

SSRIs/SNRIs

The mainstays of maintenance medical treatment in social phobia are the selective serotonin reuptake inhibitors (SSRIs) [9]. They are useful drugs for long-term therapy. Paroxetine (Paxil, Paxil CR) and sertraline (Zoloft) are approved by the U.S. Food and Drug Administration (FDA) for use in patients who suffer from social anxiety disorder. Other SSRIs are useful as well [5]. The recommendation is usually to start with a low dose of an SSRI and gradually increase to the point of symptom control, intolerance to side effects, or achievement of maximum recommended dosage. The SSRIs are normally well-tolerated medications with a low occurrence of serious side effects and minimal toxicity. Unless there is coexistent panic disorder, patients with SAD do not seem to be as likely to develop hyperstimulation effects during initiation of SSRIs; therefore, staring at very low doses is not always necessary.

Venlafaxine extended release (Effexor XR) is a serotonin-norepinephrine reuptake inhibitor (SNRI). Effexor XR is approved by the FDA for the treatment of social anxiety disorder. Duloxetine (Cymbalta) is an SNRI that is indicated for major depression and diabetic peripheral neuropathic pain. Cymbalta is not approved by the FDA for use in social anxiety disorder. Although no studies exist for the use of Cymbalta in this disorder, there are reports suggesting its potential use in the future (Table 9.1) [10].

Benzodiazepines

The benzodiazepine class of medications can be helpful in the pharmacological treatment of social anxiety disorder [5,8]. The more commonly used benzodiazepines are the shorter-acting preparations. These include alprazolam (Xanax) and lorazepam (Ativan). Clonazepam (Klonopin) is an intermediate-acting benzodiazepine that can be helpful as well. These medications work quickly to alleviate the symptoms of anxiety and have a calming,

TABLE 9.1. Selective serotonin reuptake inhibitor/serotonin-norepinephrine reuptake inhibitor medications for use in social anxiety disorder

Medication (trade name)	Dosages available	Starting dose	Maximum dose
Paroxetine (Paxil)	10, 20, 30, 40 mg	10 mg/day	60 mg/day
Paroxetine controlled-release (Paxil CR)	12.5, 25, 37.5 mg	12.5 mg/day	37.5 mg/day
Sertraline (Zoloft)	25, 50, 100 mg	25 mg/day	200 mg/day
Venlafaxine extended-release (Effexor XR)	37.5, 75, 150 mg	37.5 mg/day	225 mg/day

Adapted from ref. [9].

TABLE 9.2. Benzodiazepines

Drug name (trade name)	Dosage supplied	Onset	Half-life	Starting dosage
Alprazolam (Xanax)	0.25 mg 0.5 mg 1 mg	15–30 minutes	12 hours	0.25–0.5 mg b.i.d.
Lorazepam (Ativan)	0.5 mg 1 mg 2 mg	15–30 minutes	14 hours	0.5 mg b.i.d.
Clonazepam (Klonopin)	0.5 mg 1 mg 2 mg	30–60 minutes	25 hours	0.5 mg b.i.d.

Adapted from refs. [5] and [8].

sedating effect. The effect of shorter-acting benzodiazepines usually last less than 8 to 12 hours. The benzodiazepines carry a risk of physical dependence when used regularly in higher doses over a long period of time. The patient may experience withdrawal symptoms of nervousness, nausea, flushing, restlessness, agitation, tachycardia, or seizure upon abrupt cessation of long-term treatment. Withdrawal symptoms may be significantly reduced or eliminated by slow tapering of the daily dose over several weeks. Physical dependence may be avoided by intermittent (prn) use (Table 9.2).

Other Pharmacological Therapy

Beta-Blockers

Beta-blockers may be helpful in episodic treatment of social anxiety disorder [5,8]. Commonly used beta-blockers are propranolol (Inderal), atenolol (Tenormin), and nadolol (Corgard). These drugs affect the adrenergic nervous system and serve to block the peripheral effects of norepinephrine and epinephrine secreted by the adrenal medulla in times of stress and anxiety. Usually, 20 mg of propranolol or 25 mg of atenolol taken 30 minutes prior to the anticipated anxiety-inducing event will blunt the physical symptoms of social anxiety disorder.

Buspirone

Buspirone (BuSpar) is a nonbenzodiazepine that may have some use in social anxiety disorder. The FDA-approved indication for buspirone is generalized anxiety disorder and not specifically for social anxiety disorder. It may serve as an adjunct to SSRI therapy in the treatment of SAD, but may not be all that effective [5].

Atypical Antipsychotics

Other medications have been used in the treatment of social anxiety disorder. There is considerable interest in the use of the newer atypical antipsychotics as adjunctive therapy to the standard therapy listed above [10]. The practitioner should note that these drugs have not been specifically approved by the FDA for use in anxiety disorders. Olanzapine (Zyprexa) was shown to be effective in a pilot study of patients with social anxiety disorder [11]. At this time, data are limited, but the future may hold promise for use of the newer atypical antipsychotics for use in social anxiety as well as other anxiety disorders.

Tricyclic Antidepressants

For many years the tricyclic antidepressant medications have been used for the treatment of anxiety disorders including social anxiety disorder. Commonly used tricyclics include amitriptyline (Elavil), nortriptyline (Pamelor), imipramine (Tofranil), and desipramine (Norpramin). These compounds have an effect at serotonin and norepinephrine reuptake sites in the brain; however, their anticholinergic side effects of blurred vision, drowsiness, dry mouth, sedation, and constipation make them less helpful when compared to the SSRIs.

Monoamine Oxidase Inhibitors

The monoamine oxidase inhibitors (MAOIs) are a class of drugs that act by decreasing the breakdown of serotonin, norepinephrine, and dopamine, thereby increasing the effect of those neurotransmitters at the postsynaptic site. The MAOIs have proven to be effective in major depression and anxiety disorders including social anxiety disorder; however, their use has been limited due to the relative risk of serious adverse events [12]. Dietary restriction of tyramine, commonly found in wine, cheeses, and other foods, is necessary to prevent a hypertensive emergency. Many medications, including over-the-counter cough and cold preparations, must be avoided during MAOI therapy. The relative safety of the SSRIs has made the use of MAOIs less common.

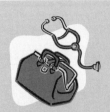

Pearls for the Practitioner

- Social anxiety disorder is a chronic problem and will usually not go in to remission by itself [6]. Keeping this in mind, the practitioner may be able to develop a long-term treatment that maintains a realistic expectation. It is always wise to discuss outcomes with the patient and avoid the perception that successful therapy is only accomplished with "pills." Often it is the unique relationship and the rapport primary care practitioners have with their patients that are the most useful tools for the treatment of SAD.

- Comorbid alcohol abuse, substance use, and depression are commonly found in patients who suffer from social anxiety disorder. The diagnosis can work both ways. A patient with alcoholism may indeed have severe social anxiety that was the stage for alcohol use in the first place (i.e., self-medication). A deeper investigation into the history of a patient with alcoholism may reveal the presence of social anxiety disorder. On the other hand, a patient who is diagnosed with SAD may have problems with alcohol that are not readily apparent upon initial presentation. A few minutes spent asking several specific questions regarding alcohol consumption or drug use may reveal additional important history.

- Whether the patient suffers from a social anxiety disorder or is exhibiting traits of avoidant personality disorder is a distinction that may seem quite blurred to the practitioner. This distinction may be difficult for the experienced psychiatrist as well. What makes the most difference in either disorder is the extent to which these conditions interfere with the patient's happiness and satisfaction. The decision to intervene with pharmacological or cognitive therapy depends on the degree of the patient's distress.

- As with many anxiety disorders, successful outcome to treatment begins with a comforting, calming, and reassuring approach from the practitioner. Many times the practitioner's empathy is as effective as a prescription medicine.

Continued

Continued

Many patients place a tremendous amount of trust in their primary care practitioner. When used properly, that trust becomes a valuable tool.

- It is not unusual to "layer" different drug classes for patients who require control of symptoms. Some patients may respond to a single drug treatment, perhaps in combination with cognitive behavioral therapy. Occasionally, a patient may need an SSRI or SRNI and a benzodiazepine taken prn. Appropriate multiple drug therapy often is necessary. The multiple drug approach could include an SSRI or SRNI, a short-acting benzodiazepine prn, and a beta-blocker prn for performance situations.

References

1. Hollander E, Simeon D. Anxiety disorders. In: Hales R, Yudofsky S, eds. Textbook of Clinical Psychiatry. Washington, DC: American Psychiatric Publishing, 2003:570–582.
2. Stein M, et al. Functional impact and health utility of anxiety disorders in primary care outpatients. Med Care 2005;43(12):1164–1170.
3. Diagnostic and Statistical Manual of Mental Disorders, 4th ed., text revision. Washington, DC: American Psychiatric Association, 2000:215–216.
4. Ballenger J. Treatment of anxiety disorders to remission. J Clin Psychiatry 2001;62(suppl 12):5–9.
5. Bruce T, Saeed S. Social anxiety disorder: a common, underrecognized mental disorder. Am Fam Physician 1999;60(8):2311–2320.
6. Westernberg H. The nature of social anxiety disorder. J Clin Psychiatry 1998;59(suppl 17):20–26.
7. Sajatovic M, Ramirez L. Rating Scales in Mental Health, 2nd ed. Hudson, OH: Lexicomp, 2003:45–52.
8. Shelton R. Anxiety disorders. In: Ebert M, Loosen P, Nurcombe B, eds. Current Diagnosis and Treatment in Psychiatry. New York: Lange Medical Books/McGraw-Hill, 2000:328–340.
9. Pollack M. Social anxiety disorder: designing a pharmacologic treatment strategy. J Clin Psychiatry 1999;60(suppl 9):20–26.
10. Chourinard G. The search for new off-label indications for antidepressant, antianxiety, antipsychotic and anticonvulsant drugs. J Psychiatry Neurosci 2006;31(3):168–176.
11. Barnett S, Kramer M, Casat C, Connor K, Davidson J. Efficacy of olanzapine in social anxiety disorder: a pilot study. J Psychopharmacol 2002;16(4):365–368.
12. Schneier F. Treatment of social phobia with antidepressants. J Clin Psychiatry 2001;62(suppl):43–48.

10
Obsessive-Compulsive Disorder

James D. Helsley

DEFINITION

Obsessive-compulsive disorder (OCD) is defined as the presence of either obsessions or compulsions. Obsessions can entail the following characteristics [1]:

- Persistent/recurrent impulses and thoughts are inappropriate and intrusive and lead to severe anxiety.
- The thoughts and impulses are beyond real-life concerns and worries.
- The patient attempts to suppress or dispense with the thoughts by creation of another thought or neutralizing action.
- The patient understands that the intrusive thoughts are generated in his/her own mind.

Compulsions can entail the following characteristics [1]:

- Repetitious behaviors or actions are performed secondary to an obsession. The act follows a scripted course without deviation.
- The behaviors and actions are performed as an avenue to prevent anxiety or to preempt a perceived future untoward event.

Obsessive-compulsive disorder usually develops in adolescence or early adulthood; 75% of cases have onset before age 30 [2]. Originally considered to be a rare disorder, OCD is estimated to have a lifetime prevalence of 2.5% [2]. It affects males and females approximately equally. It is the 10th leading cause of medical disability in the industrialized world [3].

There is a considerable body of evidence that OCD is a genetic disorder [4]. A gene abnormality is thought to lead to an increase in the neuronal cell membrane sensitivity to the excitatory action of the neurotransmitter glutamate [4].

Patients with OCD may have other comorbid psychiatric disorders. Schizophrenia, depression, panic disorder, social phobia, eating disorder, autism, and Tourette's syndrome have all been demonstrated to occur in conjunction with OCD [2].

DIAGNOSIS

Obsessions are defined as repetitive, unwanted, and intrusive thoughts that remain as a persistent feature in the minds of patients who suffer from OCD [5]. These thoughts become the cause of considerable distress to the patient.

A compulsion is a behavior that develops secondary to an obsession (5). Often the patient creates various "rules" in an attempt to deal with and control the nervousness and anxiety that accompany the obsessive thought. These behaviors lead to rituals and daily routines that tend to be rigid and inflexible, such as following a well-defined script.

Common obsessions include the following [5]:

- Fear of germs, filth, dirt or contamination
- Excessively strong aversion to bodily waste and secretions
- Fear of harming a relative or friend
- Exceptional concern with orderliness, evenness, symmetry, or exactness
- Fear of sinning or having evil thoughts
- Persistent thinking and rethinking about specific images, items, sights, and sounds
- Perpetual need for reassurance

Common compulsions include the following:

- Excessive hand-washing, tooth-brushing, flossing, showering, wearing of gloves or face mask
- Repetitively double-checking door locks, appliances, switches
- Motion rituals such as entering or leaving a room via a certain path, walking on only one side of the street, using only certain doors
- Arranging items in a particular manner and rearranging the same items when disturbed
- Counting to a certain number over and over
- Saving or hoarding otherwise unneeded items

The diagnosis of OCD is made by the history, including the symptoms and a description of behaviors. Rating scales are very helpful in support of the diagnostic impression. Scales, such as the Leyton Obsessional Inventory (LOI) and the Yale-Brown Obsessive Compulsive Scale (Y-BOCS), may be administered quickly in the primary care setting [6]. The Y-BOCS may be completed by the patient in as little as 10 minutes. It should be noted that rating scales are not "stand-alone" diagnostic instruments and must be used in conjunction with the practitioner's clinical impression. These scales may support or discount the clinical impression. The answers provided on the questionnaire may offer an opportunity for the practitioner to pursue a portion of the history in more detail.

OBSESSIVE-COMPULSIVE PERSONALITY DISORDER

Many patients with personality traits of preoccupation with neatness, orderliness, detail, and completeness may suffer from obsessive-compulsive personality disorder. The hallmarks of this disorder include the following [7]:

- Perfectionism to the point of interference with task completion
- Preoccupation with order, checklists, or organization to the point of inflexibility to change
- Tendency toward strong fiscal conservatism
- Rigidity and resistance to change in routine, environment, lifestyle
- Tendency to hoard objects
- Tendency toward inflexibility in moral, ethical, or social values
- Strong commitment to work, job performance, and productivity
- Stubbornness

While some of these personality traits may serve the patient well in certain circumstances, there may be instances where these personality features interfere with the patient's happiness, interpersonal relationships, and overall satisfaction. In some milder cases medical or psychotherapeutic intervention may not be necessary at all. The hallmark of obsessive-compulsive personality disorder is the considerable preoccupation with detail, neatness, and rigidity toward change. These patients may seem chronically unhappy and may exhibit symptoms of depression. Medical treatment may be necessary in patients who suffer from enough features of this disorder that life satisfaction and happiness are compromised.

There is obvious overlap in the features of OCD and obsessive-compulsive personality disorder. In many cases the difference is a matter of degree. Often it is difficult to make a clear distinction between the two disorders. The practitioner may find it wise to reevaluate the patient over time in order to achieve a clearer picture of the obsessive-compulsive symptoms and behaviors. Rethinking the diagnosis periodically may be very helpful to the practitioner.

TREATMENT

Cognitive Behavior Therapy

Cognitive behavior therapy (CBT) may help patients deal with the disabling behaviors and symptoms of OCD [8]. Education and insight from CBT may allow the patient who is hindered by obsessions and compulsions to cope better with their illness and make satisfactory life adjustments. Referral to a therapist experienced in OCD treatment may be a helpful strategy.

Medical Therapy

Medication has been found to be of significant help in the treatment of patients with OCD [8]. Serotonin reuptake inhibiting medications are the mainstay of pharmacological therapy in OCD [9]. The selective serotonin reuptake inhibitors (SSRIs) and tricyclic antidepressants (TCAs) have been used to treat this condition. The U.S. Food and Drug Administration (FDA) has approved the following medications for use in OCD [10]:

1. Clomipramine (Anafranil)
2. Fluoxetine (Prozac)
3. Fluvoxamine (Luvox)
4. Paroxetine (Paxil)
5. Sertraline (Zoloft)

Clomipramine (Anafranil) is a tricyclic compound that possesses potent serotonin reuptake inhibition activity. It is chemically related to other tricyclic medications, such as amitriptyline (Elavil), imipramine (Tofranil), desipramine (Norpramin), doxepin (Sinequan), and nortriptyline (Pamelor). Clomipramine is available in 25-, 50-, and 75-mg doses. The usual staring dose is 25 to 50 mg per day and the maximum is 225 mg per day. Sedation and anticholinergic side effects, such as dry mouth, constipation, and blurred vision, may be bothersome to the patient.

Fluoxetine (Prozac), fluvoxamine (Luvox), paroxetine (Paxil), and sertraline (Zoloft) are members of the SSRI class. These medications are very effective in treating OCD, are first-line treatment, and are usually well tolerated. Side effects may include nausea, weight gain, and decreased libido. Table 10.1 lists SSRI medications approved for use in the treatment of OCD [10].

Benzodiazepines

The benzodiazepines medications are not specifically indicated for the treatment of OCD. These medications are quite useful for patients who suffer from anxiety symptoms that are secondary to

TABLE 10.1. Food and Drug Administration (FDA)-approved selective serotonin reuptake inhibitor medications for use in obsessive-compulsive disorder

Medication (trade name)	Dosages available	Starting dose	Maximum dose
Paroxetine (Paxil)	10, 20, 30, 40 mg	10 mg/day	60 mg/day
Fluoxetine (Prozac)	10, 20, 40 mg	10 mg/day	80 mg/day
Sertraline (Zoloft)	25, 50, 100 mg	25 mg/day	200 mg/day
Fluvoxamine (Luvox)	50, 100 mg	50 mg/day	300 mg/day

Adapted from ref. [9].

OCD. The shorter acting benzodiazepines are generally considered more useful and have less of a tendency to accumulate in the body. The as-needed (prn) use of a relatively small dose of alprazolam (0.25 to 0.5 mg b.i.d.) or lorazepam (0.5 to 1 mg b.i.d.) may provide anxiety symptom relief for the OCD patient. These medications serve as useful adjuncts with SSRIs for this disorder.

Shorter-acting benzodiazepines include the following:

- Alprazolam (Xanax, Xanax XR)
- Lorazepam (Ativan)
- Clonazepam (Klonopin)
- Oxazepam (Serax)

Longer-acting benzodiazepines include the following:

- Chlordiazepoxide Librium)
- Diazepam (Valium)
- Clorazepate (Tranxene)

Newer Therapeutic Approaches

Evidence from various scientific studies indicates that adding newer medications to the treatment regimen may have therapeutic advantages in some patients with OCD. Risperidone (Risperdal), olanzapine (Zyprexa), and quetiapine (Seroquel) have been used as augmentation therapy to SSRI treatment in OCD patients [11]. The newer atypical antipsychotic medications have been used in conjunction with standard antidepressant treatment in major depression as well [11]. Although not formally indicated by the FDA, they may be helpful in the treatment, especially refractory cases. Further research is needed to gather enough clinical evidence to support an FDA indication.

Topiramate (Topamax), a drug used for epilepsy and the prevention of migraine headaches, has been reported to help augment SSRI therapy in OCD [11]. While the use of newer agents is still under investigation, the future of OCD therapy may not necessarily resemble the treatment standards of today.

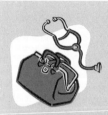

Pearls for the Practitioner

- The practitioner should develop a rapport with the patient who has OCD in an effort to gain the patient's confidence and respect. The burden of suffering from OCD is great. Many OCD patients may feel threatened by ceding control of their care to the practitioner. The patient may incorrectly, but understandably, see a visit to the practitioner as a form of defeat rather than an avenue to receive help. This may be an appropriate time for the practitioner to educate and reassure the patient regarding their illness. It may be wise to reassure the patient that treatment of OCD is collaborative, not adversarial. The OCD patient may have an intense fear of losing control. The practitioner must recognize that this fear may drive a lot of the patient's behavior. Once the patient's emotions are validated by the practitioner, the way is cleared to a more successful therapy.

- It is likely that a patient who suffers from OCD will also suffer from other mental health problems including major depression, social anxiety, panic disorder, bipolar disorder, and personality disorders. Different medications are often required for different comorbid conditions. A general rule of thumb is to treat the most pressing diagnosis first, then add or adjust medications as treatment progresses.

- Some patients with OCD may perceive that their condition is not an illness at all and requires no intervention or treatment. This poses a difficult problem for the practitioner particularly if the symptoms are severe. It is often helpful to enlist the assistance of a therapist, trusted family members, or seek a consultation with a psychiatrist to deal with this event.

- The SSRIs are the main source of treatment for OCD patients. These medications are usually well tolerated. On occasion, a patient may discontinue medication therapy without informing the practitioner. Reasons for discontinuation may include affordability, side effects, "control" issues, and the stigma of taking an antidepressant. Reviewing treatment medications and dosages at each visit is helpful in making certain the patient is maintaining therapy.

References

1. Obsessive-compulsive disorder. In: American Psychiatric Association. Diagnostic and Statistical Manual of Mental Disorders, 4th ed., text revision (DSM-IV-TR). Arlington, VA: American Psychiatric Publishing, 2000:217–218.
2. Hollander E, Simeon D. Anxiety disorders. In: Hales R, Yudofsky S, eds. Textbook of Clinical Psychiatry. Washington, DC: American Psychiatric Publishing, 2003:582–595.
3. Eisen J, et al. Impact of obsessive-compulsive disorder on quality of life. Compr Psychiatry 2006;47(4):270–275.
4. Leckman J, Kim Y. A primary candidate gene for obsessive-compulsive disorder. Arch Gen Psychiatry 2006;63:717–720.
5. Information from your family doctor. Am Fam Physician 2000;61(5):1523–1543.
6. Sajatovic M, Ramierez L. Rating Scales in Mental Health. Hudson, OH: Lexi-Comp 2003:53–60.
7. Obsessive-compulsive personality disorder. In: American Psychiatric Association. Diagnostic and Statistical Manual of Mental Disorders, 4th ed., text revision (DSM-IV-TR). Arlington, VA: American Psychiatric Publishing, 2000:296–297.
8. Soomro G. Obsessive-compulsive disorder. In: Tovey D, ed. dir. Clinical Evidence. London: BMJ Publishing Group, 2005:337–339.
9. Denys D. Pharmacotherapy of obsessive-compulsive disorder and obsessive-compulsive spectrum disorders. Psychiatric Clin North Am 2006;29(2):553–584.
10. DeBattista C, Schatzberg A. Psychotropic dosing and monitoring guidelines. Primary Psychiatry 2003;10(7):80–96.
11. Rasmussen K. Creating more effective antidepressants: clues from the clinic. Drug Discovery Today 2006;11(13/14):623–631.
12. Hollander E, Dell'Osso B. Topiramate plus paroxetine in treatment-resistant obsessive-compulsive disorder. Int Clin Psychopharmacol 2006;21(3):189–191.

.

11
Posttraumatic Stress Disorder

James D. Helsley

Primary care practitioners are increasingly being called upon by patients to treat mental disorders [1]. Included in the mix of psychiatric illnesses that a primary care practitioner may encounter is posttraumatic stress disorder (PTSD). Although described in early Greek history, it was not until 1980 that the term was accepted as an official diagnosis in the *Diagnostic and Statistical Manual of Mental Disorders,* 3rd edition (DSM-III) [2]. Terms such as "shell shock" and "flashback" have been used in the past to describe the effect of war-related experiences from World War I and II [2,3]. The lasting effect of PTSD on the lives of those afflicted can be disabling.

DEFINITION
The *Diagnostic and Statistical Manual of Mental Disorders,* 4th edition, text revision (DSM-IV-TR) has established criteria for the diagnosis of PTSD. Table 11.1 lists the features necessary for the clinician to arrive at the PTSD diagnosis. Three general features of PTSD have been described [3]: [1] persistent recollections and reexperiences, [2] avoidance of situations that might prompt a reexperience of the prior traumatic event, and [3] increased arousal and hypervigilance.

Dissociative states, periods of haziness, surreal surroundings, and distortion of time may occur in patients suffering from PTSD [5]. The patient may experience emotional desensitization with decreased response to the environment, friends, and family [5]. This may lead to emotional detachment and loss of interest. The patient may also experience symptoms of autonomic arousal, hyperactivity, irritability, and sleep disturbance [5].

COMORBIDITY
There tends to be a significantly higher incidence of comorbid psychiatric illnesses in patients with PTSD. Studies have found coexistent disorders in as many as 62% to 99% of patients [6]. Table 11.2 lists some comorbid psychiatric conditions in patients with PTSD.

TABLE 11.1. Diagnostic criteria for posttraumatic stress disorder

The patient must have been exposed to a traumatic event during which
   the patient experienced or witnessed serious injury, death, or a severe
   threat to well-being.
The patient's response was one of intense fear and horror.
The patient continues to reexperience vivid, intrusive, and disturbing
   images or thoughts.
The reexperience may involve dreams.
The patient senses a recurring feeling that the traumatic event is about
   to imminently recur.
There may be certain symbolic cues that cause the patient to develop
   distress and anxiety including physiological responses.
The patient seeks sanctuary from stimuli that evoke the reexperience and
   will avoid encounters, activities, or situations that may lead to distress.
There may be withdrawal from others and a feeling of detachment from
   friends and family.
The patient may perceive that "normal" life is not a future possibility.
Insomnia, sleep disturbances, anxiety symptoms, and an increased startle
   response may occur.
The duration of symptoms is greater than 1 month and causes significant
   distress and impairment.

Adapted from ref. [4].

TABLE 11.2. Common comorbid psychiatric illnesses in posttraumatic stress
disorder

Major depression
Phobias and other anxiety disorders
Substance use disorders (alcohol, drugs)
Personality disorders (antisocial, borderline)
Conduct disorder

Adapted from ref. [6].

In some older patients with PTSD, medical illness may develop
as a comorbid event. Studies of male veterans found a greater
incidence of diabetes mellitus, heart disease, obesity, and osteoar-
thritis in patients with PTSD [3].

The lifetime prevalence for PTSD has been reported to be
as high as 7.8% [7]. Besides psychiatric comorbidities, other
factors may play a role in determining whether or not a traumatic event leads to PTSD. The type of trauma (e.g., a natural
vs. man-made traumatic event), the patient's natural resiliency,

genetic predisposition, and experience with other past traumas may have an impact on the development of PTSD together or individually [7].

NEUROBIOLOGY

Studies have demonstrated changes in neurological and biological function in patients suffering from PTSD. Low plasma γ-aminobutyric acid (GABA) levels have been found in patients diagnosed with PTSD secondary to motor vehicle accidents [8]. It is postulated that lower levels of GABA may predispose to the development of PTSD. Allopregnenolone and pregnenolone have a modulating effect on GABA receptors. Low levels of allopregnenolone have been found in women who suffer from PTSD [9]. The lower levels of these modulators are postulated to allow for greater neural excitatory activity. This may also play a role in reexperiencing type symptoms [9].

Measurement of cortisol levels in PTSD patients did not demonstrate any difference between PTSD and normal patients [10]. This finding supports the conclusion that there is no adrenal cortical "biological" stress response in PTSD [10].

Brain structural abnormalities have been demonstrated in patients with PTSD. Magnetic resonance imaging methodology has demonstrated changes in hippocampus and amygdala volume in some patients with PTSD [11].

It is most likely that the development of PTSD is a result of multiple, complex anatomical and neurobiological factors in patients who may have an existing predisposition. Other psychological and social issues would also be expected to play a role in PTSD development.

ACUTE STRESS DISORDER

Acute stress disorder (ASD) is a phenomenon with similar symptoms and features of PTSD; however, the onset of the disorder occurs within 1 month following exposure of the triggering traumatic event [4]. Upon experiencing a traumatic event the patient may develop a sense of numbing, emotional detachment, depersonalization, or dissociative amnesia. The traumatic event may then go on to be persistently reexperienced. Considerable anxiety may develop, and the patient may exhibit avoidance behavior in order to prevent situations that might trigger a reexperience. Increased arousal may be present. The above symptoms combine to produce impairment of adequate functioning and interfere with overall happiness and satisfaction.

TREATMENT

The treatment of PTSD and ASD centers on therapeutic approaches that include the control of symptoms, prevention of relapse, restoration of adequate function, and limitation of comorbid conditions [12]. The three most widely recognized interventions are as follows:

1. Psychopharmacology (medication)
2. Psychotherapeutic interventions (e.g., cognitive behavior therapy and other types of psychotherapy)
3. Psychoeducation

Psychopharmacology

The selective serotonin reuptake inhibitors (SSRIs) are considered the first-line treatment for patients with PTSD [12,13]. These medications are effective in improving the quality of life in patients with PTSD as well as in the treatment of comorbid conditions such as depression, panic disorder, social phobia, and obsessive-compulsive disorder [12,13]. Table 11.3 lists the two SSRIs currently approved by the U.S. Food and Drug Administration (FDA) for use in PTSD.

Improvement in patients with PTSD has also been demonstrated with the use of fluoxetine (Prozac) [13]. Venlafaxine (Effexor XR), a serotonin-norepinephrine reuptake inhibitor (SNRI) has also been shown to be effective in PTSD [14].

The newer atypical antipsychotic medications have shown promise in the treatment of PTSD. Studies using olanzapine (Zyprexa), quetiapine (Seroquel), and risperidone (Risperdal) have demonstrated effectiveness particularly when psychotic symptoms are present [12]. Further studies are needed to firmly establish the use of this class of medications in PTSD.

TABLE 11.3. Selective serotonin reuptake inhibitor medications approved by the U.S. Food and Drug Administration for use in posttraumatic stress disorder

Medication (trade name)	Dosages available	Starting dose	Maximum dose
Paroxetine (Paxil)	10, 20, 30, 40 mg	20 mg/day	40 mg/day
Sertraline (Zoloft)	25, 50, 100 mg	25 mg/day	200 mg/day

Adapted from refs. [12] and [13].

Tricyclic antidepressants (amitriptyline and imipramine) have been shown to have efficacy in the treatment of PTSD [12]. The studies investigating the use of the tricyclics were mostly in combat veterans, which may limit the extrapolation for their use in the general population.

Benzodiazepines have been used successfully in a variety of anxiety disorders. The use of benzodiazepines in PTSD has not been clearly established [15]. Shorter acting benzodiazepines (alprazolam, lorazepam) may help in the short-term treatment of PTSD sleep-related problems, but long-term use is not recommended [12].

To date, beta-blockers and anticonvulsants have not been demonstrated to be effective pharmacological treatments in PTSD [12]. Future studies may add useful information regarding the use of beta-blockers in modulating the emotional and psychiatric effects of trauma.

Psychotherapeutic Interventions

Cognitive behavior therapy (CBT) has been demonstrated to be beneficial in the treatment of PTSD when compared to no treatment. Other forms of psychotherapy, hypnosis, and counseling have also been shown to be helpful [15].

Eye movement desensitization and reprocessing (EMDR) is a form of therapy that combines multiple, brief exposures to traumatic triggers with eye movement desensitization. It is used in conjunction with CBT as a therapeutic approach to patient treatment. This method has demonstrated effectiveness in PTSD [12,15]. Referral to an experienced therapist may be helpful for many patients with PTSD.

Psychoeducation and Support

Dissemination of educational material and information to a patient suffering from PTSD often provides considerable help. Besides the direct information provided, the indirect implication is that the practitioner has confidence in the patient's ability to deal with the disabling effects of PTSD. This in itself may be of considerable reassurance to the patient. Patient awareness of the symptoms of the illness and the planned therapeutic interventions will likely produce a better outcome.

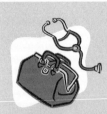

Pearls for the Practitioner

- The primary care practitioner is usually the first person who a patient with PTSD or ASD will seek for treatment. A comforting, empathetic approach is always a good starting place in the initiation of therapy. Often a simple validation of the patient's emotional reaction and symptoms is all that is necessary to effect adequate treatment.
- Some practitioners may feel comfortable with their ability to provide counseling and psychoeducation for patients. Time constraints often prohibit the primary care practitioner from proceeding with more involved psychotherapy. Referral to a trained therapist is acceptable and often very effective.
- Some patients with PTSD may present with other mental disorders such as phobias, panic attacks, and depression. The practitioner may find it useful to take a few extra minutes and ask for details of a prior traumatic event because the patient may be embarrassed or reluctant to openly offer important historical information. The extra time spent early in the diagnosis and treatment of PTSD will likely yield a better long-term result for both patient and practitioner.
- As neuroimaging techniques improve in the future, the practitioner may have objective ways to determine the effect of a traumatic event on the brain.
- The use of beta-blockade in the future treatment of PTSD may become of significant value. Once thought to be of no value, beta-blockers have been demonstrated to modulate norepinephrine activity in the amygdala of fear-conditioned rats (16).

References

1. Daly R. Primary Care Treating More Serious Mental illness. Psychiatric News 2006;41(14):7.
2. Lowe B, Henningson P, Herzog W. Posttraumatic stress disorder: history of a politically unwanted diagnosis. Psychother Psychosom Med Psychol 2006;56(3–4):182–187.

3. Vieweg W, et al. Posttraumatic stress disorder: clinical features, pathophysiology, and treatment. Am J Med 2006;119(5):383–390.

4. Posttraumatic stress disorder. Diagnostic and Statistical Manual of Mental Disorders, 4th ed., text revision (DSM-IV-TR). Arlington, VA: American Psychiatric Publishing, 2000:218–220.

5. Hollander E, Simeon D. Anxiety disorders. In: Hales R, Yudofsky S, eds. Textbook of Clinical Psychiatry, 4th ed. Washington, DC: American Psychiatric Publishing, 2003:595–607.

6. Gillette G, Fielstein E. Posttraumatic stress disorder and acute stress disorder. In: Ebert M, Loosen P, Nurcombe B, ed. Current Diagnosis and Treatment Psychiatry. New York: McGraw-Hill, 2000:341–350.

7. Matthews A, Mossefin C. The "date" that changed her life. Current Psychiatry 2006;5(2):75–87.

8. Vaiva G, Thomas P, et al. Low posttrauma GABA plasma levels as a predictive factor in the development of acute posttraumatic stress disorder. Biol Psychiatry 2004;55(3):250–254.

9. Rasmusson A, Pinna G, et al. Decreased cerebrospinal fluid allopregnanolone levels in women with posttraumatic stress disorder. Biol Psychiatry 2006;60(7):704–713.

10. Wheler G, Brandon D, et al. Cortisol production rate in posttraumatic stress disorder. J Clin Endocrinol Metab 2006;91(9):3486–3489.

11. Karl A, Schafer M, Malta L, Dorfel D, Rohleder N, Werner A. A meta-analysis of structural brain abnormalities in PTSD. Neurosci Biobehav Rev 2006;30(7):1004–1031.

12. Ursano R, et al. Practice guideline for the treatment of patients with acute stress disorder and posttraumatic stress disorder. Am J Psychiatry 2004;161(11 suppl):1–31.

13. Davis L, Frazier E, Williford R, Newell J. Long-term pharmacotherapy for posttraumatic stress disorder. CNS Drugs 2006;20(6):465–476.

14. Davidson J, Rothbaum B, Tucker P, Asnis G, Benattia I, Musgung J. Venlafaxine-extended release in posttraumatic stress disorder: a sertraline and placebo controlled study. J Clin Psychopharmacology 2006;26(3):259–267.

15. Bisson J. Posttraumatic stress disorder In: Clinical Evidence Concise, vol. 15. London: BMJ Publishing Group, 2006:379–382.

16. Debeic J, LeDoux J. Noradrenergic signaling in the amygdala contributes to the reconsolidation of fear memory: treatment implications for PTSD. Ann NY Acad Sci 2006;1071:521–524.

12
Generalized Anxiety Disorder

James D. Helsley

Every person experiences anxiety at times throughout life. It may be considered a normal part of development. The experience gained by dealing with life's episodes of anxiety can help a person deal with subsequent anxiety-provoking situations in the future; however, for some, anxiety may become persistent, unrelenting, and disabling.

Generalized anxiety disorder (GAD) has been estimated to occur with an incidence of about 5% of the general population. Women are affected more than men [1]. Comorbidity with major depression, other anxiety disorders, and other psychiatric disorders may be as high as 90% [1].

DEFINITION
According to the *Diagnostic and Statistical Manual of Mental Disorders*, 4th edition, text revision (DSM-IV-TR) [2] generalized anxiety disorder is defined by the following:

- Persistent, excessive worry, apprehension, and anxiety lasting at least 6 months
- Presence of three or more of the following: restlessness, fatigue, difficulty concentrating, irritability, muscle tension, insomnia, or disturbed sleep
- The patient cannot fully control the anxiety
- Absence of a specific disorder, such as panic disorder, social phobia, anorexia nervosa, posttraumatic stress disorder, separation anxiety, obsessive-compulsive disorder, hypochondriasis
- The anxiety causes significant impairment of interpersonal functioning
- The anxiousness is not a result of an external substance or medical condition
- The anxiety is not part of a mood disorder or psychotic disorder

Generalized anxiety disorder usually begins in early adulthood. It is a common disorder seen in primary care [3]. The disorder is characterized by a persistent state of worry and apprehension. There is usually an exaggerated level of "sensory alertness."

Generalized anxiety disorder is more likely to occur in patients with chronic medical illnesses, such as hypertension, diabetes mellitus, chronic obstructive pulmonary disease, and irritable bowel syndrome [4]. Personality disorders are common in patients with GAD [5].

Generalized anxiety disorder is a chronic disorder [5]. It may go unrecognized for years after its onset in early adulthood. The patient's array of somatic symptoms will often prompt the visit to the clinician. The subsequent clinical evaluation of these symptoms through diagnostic testing has led to higher health care costs in GAD patients [5].

ETIOLOGY

The underlying biological cause of GAD is not fully understood. Animal models and some clinical studies implicate the dysfunction of various neurotransmitters in the etiology of GAD [5,6]. Serotonin, norepinephrine, and γ-aminobutyric acid (GABA) dysregulation is thought to play a significant role in producing the symptoms of GAD. Genetics may also play a role. Twin studies have demonstrated similar risk factors that may predispose to GAD and depression [7]. Environmental factors, particularly a history of trauma, have also been associated with GAD [5].

Recent studies have implicated glutamate in the development of anxiety and mood disorders [8]. Glutamate is an amino acid neurotransmitter that allows for rapid synaptic neurotransmission. Theories suggest that dysregulation of glutamate in certain foci in the brain may allow for greater "rapid firing" of anxiety response pathways, leading to the series of symptoms collectively referred to as anxiety disorders [9]. To date, most treatments have centered on serotonin reuptake activity (selective serotonin reuptake inhibitors, SSRIs) and GABA activity (benzodiazepines). While these treatments are currently effective and available, the future may find the use of new medications that regulate glutamate superior in the treatment of GAD.

It appears that the final answer to the underlying cause of GAD will be multifactorial and not a single, simple, or potentially correctable cause. It follows, then, that treatment will be likely multifactorial as well.

EVALUATION

Rating Scales

The diagnostic criteria for GAD, as adapted from the DSM-IV-TR, are listed above. In addition to the clinical presentation and symptoms, the clinician may find the use of rating scales helpful in confirming the diagnosis of GAD. Several scales have been published. Table 12.1 lists some of the more common anxiety rating scales [10, 11]. These scales are brief and can be administered quickly by the practitioner. The most popular scale is the Hamilton Rating Scale for Anxiety. It is designed to aid in the initial assessment, as well as to monitor changes in anxiety levels over time. Note that none of the rating scales is absolute, and none should be used as a stand-alone criterion for the diagnosis of GAD.

Medical Disorders

Before GAD can be fully diagnosed, medical disorders should be considered as causes of anxiety symptoms. Hyperthyroidism, carcinoid syndrome, pheochromocytoma, Cushing's disease, and mitral valve prolapse may all present with symptoms of anxiety as prominent features [4]. Heart disease, anemia, hypoglycemia, menopause, seizure disorder, asthma, chronic obstructive pulmonary disease, vertigo, and central nervous system (CNS) diseases may all have anxiety-like symptomatology [12]. Significant medical disorders usually have other symptoms and clinical findings that are obvious and preclude the diagnosis of GAD. On occasion, the practitioner may wish to proceed with a medical workup. Generally, a complete blood count, glucose, chemistry panel, urinalysis, and thyroid-stimulating hormone level make up a modest-cost battery of tests that suffices to establish (or eliminate) the diagnosis of a medical disorder. Neuroimaging studies, electroen-

TABLE 12.1. Clinical rating scales for general anxiety disorder

Scale name	Number of questions	Completion time required
Hamilton Rating Scale for Anxiety (HAM-A)	14	20 minutes
Covi Anxiety Scale (COVI)	3	5–10 minutes
Sheehan Disability Scale	3	Less than 5 minutes
State-Trait Anxiety Inventory (STAI)	4	10 minutes
GAD-7 Scale	7	5 minutes

Adapted from refs. [10] and [11].

cephalogram (EEG), specialty referral, and more involved laboratory investigation should be reserved for cases where the history and physical findings warrant more in-depth study.

Substance Abuse
Nicotine and caffeine are commonly used stimulant substances that produce side effects that may resemble anxiety. Alcohol withdrawal and withdrawal from addictive substances (narcotics, high-dose benzodiazepines, barbiturates) can produce significant anxiety symptoms. A careful history for substance use is very important in the evaluation of patients with symptoms of anxiety.

Comorbidity
Generalized anxiety disorder is commonly a comorbid feature with other psychiatric disorders. Major depression, bipolar disorder, panic disorder, substance abuse, dysthymia, or other anxiety disorders may frequently be encountered in a patient with symptoms of GAD [13].

Major depression is the most common comorbid condition in GAD, occurring in two thirds of patients [13]. Generalized anxiety disorder symptoms may occur at any time during the course of major depression [4]. An anxious patient may suffer from significant depression and vice versa.

TREATMENT
The goal of therapy in GAD is to achieve remission [14]. Many patients with GAD are considered to be incompletely treated, which prompts the need for improvements in awareness, diagnosis, and treatment [14]. Successful treatment often requires a multifaceted approach that takes into consideration psychiatric, medical, emotional, financial, cultural, and social issues. Often the primary care practitioner is in a unique position to have a full understanding of these issues for many patients. This knowledge enables the practitioner to proceed with treatment in an effective and efficient manner.

Cognitive Behavior Therapy
Cognitive behavior therapy (CBT) is a useful and helpful treatment for GAD [15]. The aim of CBT is to ameliorate the symptoms of GAD by helping patients deal with basic fears and uncertainties that lead to overwhelming anxiety. Education and enhanced awareness may allow some patients to come to grips with their disorder. The components of CBT include techniques of relaxation, increased awareness, and education. The following techniques of CBT are useful in the treatment of GAD [15]:

- Applied relaxation
- Education about GAD etiology and what the symptoms represent
- Cognitive restructuring
- Increased awareness of self
- Understanding and monitoring anxiety symptoms and their relationship to somatic sensations
- Learning to cope with and modify automatic reactions to known anxiety-inducing stimuli

Cognitive behavior therapy is usually managed best by someone trained in the fields of psychology and counseling. Group therapy may be useful in some cases. Therapy may require up to 4 months to complete [15].

Pharmacotherapy

The pharmacological treatment of GAD is divided into several different classes of medication. The following review addresses some of the more common medications used in general clinical practice:

Benzodiazepines

The benzodiazepine class of medication is very effective in treating the symptoms of GAD [16]. These drugs work by enhancing the effects of GABA and hence decreasing the degree of neuronal discharge in the locus ceruleus [16]. Table 12.2 lists the benzodiazepines that are commonly used for patients with GAD.

Selective Serotonin Reuptake Inhibitors

Currently, paroxetine (Paxil) and escitalopram (Lexapro) are the only two SSRIs approved by the U.S. Food and Drug Administration (FDA) for use in GAD. The other SSRI medications have various

TABLE 12.2. Benzodiazepines for generalized anxiety disorder (GAD)

Drug name	Dosage supplied	Onset	Half-life	Starting dosage
Alprazolam (Xanax)	0.25 mg 0.5 mg 1 mg	15–30 minutes	12 hours	0.25–0.5 mg b.i.d.
Lorazepam (Ativan)	0.5 mg 1 mg 2 mg	15–30 minutes	14 hours	0.5 mg b.i.d.
Clonazepam (Klonopin)	0.5 mg 1 mg 2 mg	30–60 minutes	25 hours	0.5 mg b.i.d.

Adapted from ref. [16].

FDA indication approvals that include major depression and other specific anxiety disorders. The International Consensus Group on Depression and Anxiety recommends an SSRI as first-line therapy in depression or any of the anxiety disorders [17]. Any of the currently available SSRIs would likely be beneficial in the treatment of GAD. For example, studies of sertraline (Zoloft) have shown it to be effective in GAD patients [18].

In general, initiation of SSRI treatment should begin at lower doses (compared to initial treatment of depression) in order to minimize side effects. After initiation of therapy, the dose of SSRI may be advanced over the ensuing 4 to 12 weeks to achieve optimal results [19].

Common side effects of the SSRIs include nausea, headache, muscle tension, restlessness, decreased libido, delayed ejaculation, anorgasmia, sedation, weight gain, diarrhea, vivid dreams, rash, and increased sweating [19]. Some side effects are dose related. Side effects are usually relatively mild, do not prompt discontinuation, and tend to fade as treatment progresses.

Table 12.3 lists some SSRIs useful in the treatment of GAD.

TABLE 12.3. Selective serotonin reuptake inhibitor medications useful in the treatment of generalized anxiety disorder

Drug name (trade name)	Dosage supplied	Maximum dosage/day	Half-life dosage	Starting
Escitalopram (Lexapro) FDA approved	5 mg 10 mg 20 mg	40 mg	30 hours	5 mg q.d.
Paroxetine (Paxil) FDA approved	10 mg 20 mg 30 mg 40 mg	60 mg	21 hours	10 mg q.d.
Citalopram (Celexa)	10 mg 20 mg 40 mg	60 mg	35 hours	10 mg q.d.
Paroxetine (Paxil CR)	12.5 mg 25 mg 37.5 mg	75 mg	21 hours	12.5 mg q.d.
Sertraline (Zoloft)	25 mg 50 mg 100 mg	200 mg	25 hours	25 mg q.d.
Fluoxetine (Prozac)	10 mg 20 mg 40 mg	80 mg	4–6 days	10 mg q.d.

CR, controlled release; FDA, U.S. Food and Drug Administration. Adapted from ref. [17].

Buspirone

Buspirone (BuSpar) is approved by the FDA for the treatment of GAD. Buspirone is a nonbenzodiazepine that acts as a partial agonist at postsynaptic serotonin receptors in the hippocampus [15]. The full effect of buspirone may not be seen for several weeks after initiation of therapy [4]. Side effects include nausea and dizziness. Dosing usually begins with 5 mg three times daily (t.i.d.) and may be advanced up to 20 mg t.i.d. The delayed response and t.i.d. dosing schedule make buspirone a less attractive option for the treatment of GAD.

Serotonin-Norepinephrine Reuptake Inhibitors

The serotonin-norepinephrine reuptake inhibitor (SNRI) medications include venlafaxine (Effexor, Effexor XR) and duloxetine (Cymbalta). Venlafaxine, in its extended release form (Effexor XR), is approved by the FDA for use in patients with GAD. Duloxetine is approved by the FDA for use in major depression, neuropathic pain, and generalized anxiety disorder. Because both venlafaxine and duloxetine have action on serotonin reuptake, they would be expected to have benefit in the treatment of both depression and anxiety. Duloxetine has been found to be effective in treating the symptoms of anxiety [20]. It is very likely that the SNRIs are as effective as the SSRIs in the treatment of anxiety disorders [21].

The starting dose for venlafaxine extended-release (Effexor XR) is 37.5 mg once a day. The dose may be titrated up to 225 mg daily [15]. Onset of action begins about 2 weeks after initiation of therapy. Side effects include nausea, sweating, dry mouth, blurred vision, and sexual dysfunction [15].

Duloxetine may be started at 20 or 30 mg once daily and advanced to 60 mg once daily depending upon response. The maximum daily dose of duloxetine for the treatment of GAD is 120 mg. Duloxetine may also be started at the 60 mg once-daily dose and maintained thereafter [20]. Initiation of therapy with the 60-mg dose may produce side effects or worsen anxiety symptoms. The practitioner is cautioned to use lower starting doses for duloxetine when treating anxiety disorders.

Tricyclic Antidepressants

In years past, the tricyclic antidepressants (TCAs) were found to be useful in treatment of anxiety disorders, as well as major depression. Side effects and potential toxicity have made their use less favorable than the SSRIs. Dry mouth, sedation, constipation, orthostatic hypotension, and weight gain are considerable side effects of TCAs. Because of this unfavorable side-effect profile, their use is not considered a first-line option in the treatment of

GAD [15]. Commonly prescribed TCAs are amitriptyline (Elavil), nortriptyline (Pamelor), clomipramine (Anafranil), imipramine (Tofranil), and desipramine (Norpramin).

Monoamine Oxidase Inhibitors

Monamine oxidase inhibitors (MAOIs) are compounds that have been used for the treatment of depression and anxiety [1]. These medications are usually reserved for refractory patients who do not respond adequately to trials of other antidepressant therapy [1]. Use of MAOIs involves therapeutic problems, the most prominent of which is the need to restrict dietary tyramine. In the presence of an MAOI, tyramine, which is found in cheese, sauerkraut, fermented products, and aged foods, can produce a severe hypertensive crisis [22]. Patients must be warned about this potential problem and given a list of foods to avoid while on MAOI treatment. The patient must also be cautioned about other medications that may negatively interact with MAOIs, such as cough and cold preparations and other antidepressants.

Other Treatments

- Beta-blockers have potential use in GAD, particularly in helping to control tremor and other physiological effects of the anxiety disorder [4]. Common beta-blockers are propranolol (Inderal), nadolol (Corgard), metoprolol (Lopressor), and atenolol (Tenormin).
- Antihistamines possess sedating side effects that may be of value in treating GAD; however, these medications are not considered very effective [4]. Common antihistamines include hydroxyzine (Vistaril), diphenhydramine (Benadryl), and meclizine (Antivert). These medications have no significant role in GAD treatment.
- Exercise has been thought by some to help in the treatment of anxiety disorders. A review of 11 trials involving the use of exercise as treatment for anxiety in children and adolescents showed no significant difference in exercise-treated groups [23]. Exercise may have modest effect on depression in this age group [23].
- There has been recent interest in the use of the newer atypical antipsychotic medications in the treatment of anxiety disorders. Studies have been conducted using risperidone (Risperdal), olanzapine (Zyprexa), quetiapine (Seroquel), and aripiprazole (Abilify) in conjunction with various SSRIs in the treatment of disorders including GAD, panic disorder, obsessive-compulsive disorder, and major depression [24]. Most of the studies report improvement in

symptoms of the disorder studied. The practitioner should note that the use of the atypical antipsychotic medications in the treatment of GAD is not currently approved by the U.S. Food and Drug Administration. Perhaps increased knowledge of the usefulness of these agents will be gained in the future.

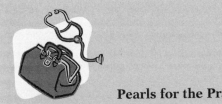

Pearls for the Practitioner

- The use of rating scales is important in the diagnosis of GAD. Although rating scales are helpful, they are not intended to be a substitute for the practitioner's clinical impression. The practitioner may find it useful to become familiar with one or two of the scales and use them as a regular part of the evaluation. Familiarity with a particular scale allows for a more efficient patient evaluation.
- Psychiatric evaluation and diagnosis is primarily a clinical process based on history and patient presentation. Compared to the rest of clinical medicine, there are few diagnostic tests for the practitioner to employ when making a psychiatric diagnosis. Many patients have become accustomed to the use of scans, x-rays, and blood tests. A rating scale may be viewed by the patient as a "test." For this reason, use of a rating scale may help add validity to the practitioner's clinical impression and allow for greater patient acceptance of recommended treatment.
- The issue of when to refer a patient with psychiatric illness is a common problem. Many primary care practitioners are quite comfortable and do an admirable job in treating a broad range of mental health conditions. Other practitioner's are less comfortable. In general, referral for consultation to a psychiatrist is a matter of individual discretion. If the patient is tolerating therapy and is improving, the practitioner may wish to continue treatment and make adjustments as needed. If the patient fails to respond to treatment, appears suicidal, experiences untoward side effects, or is not responding as anticipated, the practitioner may wish to refer.

References

1. Hollander E, Simeon D. Anxiety disorders. In: Hales R, Yudofsky S, eds. Textbook of Clinical Psychiatry, 4th ed. Washington, DC: American Psychiatric Publishing, 2003:543–630.
2. American Psychiatric Association. Diagnostic and Statistical Manual of Mental Disorders, 4th ed., text revision (DSM-IV-TR). Arlington, VA: American Psychiatric Publishing, 2000:222–223.
3. Shelton R. Anxiety disorders. In: Ebert M, Loosen P, Nurcombe B, eds. Current Diagnosis and Treatment in Psychiatry. New York: McGraw-Hill, 2000:328–340.
4. Gliatto M. Generalized anxiety disorder. Am Fam Physician 2000;62(7): 1501–1502.
5. Kniele K, Brawman-Mintzer O. Diagnosis and treatment of generalized anxiety disorder. CNS News 2006;8(7):17–23.
6. Jetty P, Charney D, Goddard A. Neurobiology of generalized anxiety disorder. Psychiatric Clin North Am 2001;24(1):75–97.
7. Kendler K. Reflections on the relationship between psychiatric genetics and psychiatric nosology. Am J Psychiatry 2006;163(7):1138–1146.
8. Mathew S. Glutamate modulation in mood and anxiety disorders: toward a rational pharmacology? CNS Spectrums 2005;10(10):806–807.
9. Cortese B, Phan K. The role of glutamate in anxiety and related disorders. CNS Spectrums 2005;10(10):820–830.
10. Spitzer R, Kroeneke K, Williams J, Lowe B. A brief measure for assessing generalized anxiety disorder: the GAD-7. Arch Intern Med 2006;166(10):1092–1097.
11. Sajatovic M, Ramirez L. Rating Scales in Mental Health, 2nd ed. Hudson, OH: Lexi-Comp, 2003:36–44.
12. Chan P, Thomas D, McKinley E, Stanford E. Outpatient and Primary Care Medicine. Laguna Hills, CA: Current Clinical Strategies Publishing, 2005:233–255.
13. Pollack M. Comorbid anxiety and depression. J Clin Psychiatry 2005;66(suppl 8):22–29.
14. Ninan P. Dissolving the burden of generalized anxiety disorder. J Clin Psychiatry 2001:62(suppl 19):5–10.
15. Rynn M, Brawman-Mintzer O. Generalized anxiety disorder: acute and chronic treatment. CNS Spectrums 2004;9(10):716–723.
16. Ballenger J. Overview of different pharmacotherapies for attaining remission in generalized anxiety disorder. J Clin Psychiatry 2001;62(suppl 19):11–19.
17. Ballenger J, et al. A proposed algorithm for the improved recognition and treatment of the depression/anxiety spectrum in primary care. J Clin Psychiatry Prim Care Companion 2001;3(2):44–52.
18. Brawman-Mintzer O, Knapp R, Rynn M, Carter R, Rickels K. Sertraline treatment for generalized anxiety disorder: a randomized, double-blind, placebo-controlled study. J Clin Psychiatry 2006;67(6):874–881.
19. Marangell L, Silver J, Goff D, Yudosfsky S. Psychopharmacology and electroconvulsive therapy. In: Hales R, Yudofsky S, ed. Textbook of

Clinical Psychiatry, 4th ed. Washington, DC: American Psychiatric Publishing, 2003:1047–1149.

20. Dunner D, et al. Duloxetine in treatment of anxiety symptoms associated with depression. Depression and Anxiety 2003;18:53–61.

21. Stahl S, Grady M, Moret C, Briley M. SNRIs: their pharmacology, clinical efficacy, and tolerability in comparison with other classes of antidepressants. CNS Spectrums 2005;10(9):732–747.

22. Loosen P, et al. Mood disorders. In: Ebert M, Loosen P, Nurcombe B, eds. Current Diagnosis and Treatment in Psychiatry. New York: McGraw-Hill, 2000:290–327.

23. Larun L, Nordheim L, Ekeland E, Hagen K, Heian F. Exercise in prevention and treatment of anxiety and depression among children and young people. Cochrane Database of Systematic Reviews 2006;3: CD004691. DOI: 10.1002/14651858.CD004691.pub2.

24. Rasmussen K. Creating more effective antidepressants: clues from the clinic. Drug Discovery Today 2006;11(13/14):623–631.

13
Anxiety Disorder Due to a General Medical Condition

James D. Helsley

Anxiety disorders are the most prevalent mental disorders in the United States. The economic burden is estimated to be nearly $50 billion annually [1]. The most common anxiety disorders are as follows:

- Generalized anxiety disorder (GAD)
- Panic disorder (PD)
- Obsessive-compulsive disorder (OCD)
- Phobias/social anxiety disorder
- Posttraumatic stress disorder (PTSD)
- Acute stress disorder
- Anxiety disorder due to a medical condition
- Anxiety disorder induced by a substance

The exact cause of the anxiety disorders is unknown. There is, however, considerable evidence that a deep brain structure, the amygdala, is intricately involved with the development of anxiety behavior. The amygdala is thought to mediate the fear response in the brain when an individual is confronted with real or perceived danger [2]. The response of the amygdala to a threat is to create the "fight or flight" response, which includes adrenal catecholamine release, increased heart rate, glycogenolysis, and shunting of blood from the gut. Theory holds that the inappropriate activation or dysregulation of the "fight or flight" response leads to autonomic discharge, which, in turn, produces the symptom complex common to many anxiety disorders.

It is frequently recognized that many medical illnesses and conditions are associated with a certain degree of anxiety. The uncertainty surrounding the experience of illness and its treatment can elicit anxiety in many patients, much of which is expected and natural. Exaggeration of the patient's symptoms, as well as a delay of diagnosis due to avoidance and denial, may both stem from illness-related anxiety.

Little is written about the overall aspect of the subject of anxiety in general medical conditions. There are some studies in the medical literature about specific medical diagnoses and the role anxiety plays in the care of those illnesses. This chapter discusses anxiety disorders and their relationship to some of the more common medical illnesses encountered in primary care.

DEFINITION

According to the *Diagnostic and Statistical Manual of Mental Disorders*, 4th edition, text revision (DSM-IV-TR), the diagnosis of an anxiety disorder due to a general medical condition requires the presence of a medical condition capable of being the origin of the anxiety symptoms [3]. The anxiety must be significant enough to cause distress and impairment of functioning [4].

Commonly seen in conjunction with the anxiety disorders is the comorbid illness of depression. There is symptom overlap in many cases of depression and anxiety. The following symptoms occur in both anxiety disorders and depression [2]:

- Difficulty concentrating
- Nausea, constipation, diarrhea
- Agitation
- Irritability
- Sleep disturbance (sleep latency, decreased sleep maintenance)
- Fatigue
- Pain (headache, back pain, abdominal pain, leg pain)

Not only are the above symptoms related to comorbid anxiety disorders and depression, they may also be part of a medical illness. A patient with an anxiety disorder has usually had anxiety symptoms for a long period of time. There may be a previous diagnosis of an anxiety disorder or other mental health problem. Symptoms of anxiety that are of recent onset and are identified as a new event for a patient can signal the presence of physiologic disease [2].

COMMON MEDICAL CONDITIONS ASSOCIATED WITH ANXIETY

Chronic Obstructive Pulmonary Disease

Chronic obstructive pulmonary disease (COPD) is a common ailment. It is estimated that about 28 million people in the United States are affected by COPD. Half of these patients may have not yet been diagnosed [5]. The primary symptoms are cough, sputum production, and shortness of breath. Anxiety and depression are commonly associated with COPD [6]. Studies have shown that breathlessness, physical impairment, reduced activities of daily living, hopelessness, and anxiety correlate with reduced quality of life in COPD patients [7]. Studies have also shown that some primary care practitioners do not address the emotional aspect of care in COPD patients [6]. This lapse is likely more a product of lack of time and resources than it is one of lack of knowledge or ability. Nevertheless, recognition and treatment of the COPD patient's symptoms of anxiety are important parts of the care of these individuals.

Asthma

Asthma is a common ailment affecting as many as 150 million people worldwide [8]. Symptoms of asthma include wheezing, cough, shortness of breath, chest discomfort, and fatigue. Asthma may be made worse by exercise, infection, pollutants, smoking, dust, and allergens. Anxiety disorders and depression are common comorbid conditions in asthma patients. Studies have shown that asthma patients who suffer from anxiety and depression experience poorer asthma control than those without anxiety and depression [8]. These same patients also report a lesser quality of life and higher bronchodilator use than control groups despite no difference in pulmonary function.

Often a patient with COPD or asthma does not require a change of medication for worsening of symptoms. After taking a careful history and performing a physical examination, the practitioner may come to the conclusion that underlying anxiety is the primary cause of a patient's symptoms. At that point, the practitioner may find that a comforting approach to the patient often helps treat anxiety symptoms. The practitioner may also judge that medical therapy of the anxiety is warranted.

Low doses of short-acting benzodiazepines may be helpful. Alprazolam (Xanax) in doses of 0.25 to 0.5 mg or lorazepam (Ativan) in doses of 0.5 to 1 mg once or twice daily may provide satisfactory anxiety symptom relief.

Use of SSRI medications in COPD and asthma patients may also provide considerable improvement in anxiety symptoms. Sertraline (Zoloft), escitalopram (Lexapro), citalopram (Celexa), paroxetine (Paxil, Paxil CR), and fluoxetine (Prozac) are all useful in the treatment of anxiety symptoms. Venlafaxine (Effexor, Effexor XR) is a serotonin-norepinephrine reuptake inhibitor (SNRI) that also may be helpful in treating anxiety due to asthma or COPD.

Medication-Related Anxiety in Chronic Obstructive Pulmonary Disease/Asthma

The medications used for the therapy of COPD and asthma may produce side effects that mimic the symptoms of anxiety or make an underlying anxiety disorder worse. The practitioner should remain alert for the possibility that anxiety symptoms in a COPD or asthma patient may not necessarily represent the diagnosis of an anxiety disorder. The symptoms may be due entirely to medication side effects. The following is a discussion of some of the more common medicines used in the treatment of COPD/asthma and their potential relationship to the symptoms of an anxiety disorder:

- Albuterol (Proventil, Ventolin) and salmeterol (Advair) are bronchodilator medications commonly used in the treatment of lung disease. Albuterol and salmeterol belong to the sympathomimetic amine class of drugs [9]. Besides the desired effect of bronchodilation, these drugs may produce increased heart rate, nervousness, tremor, insomnia, nausea, and decreased appetite. These side effects may overlap with the symptoms of an anxiety disorder.
- Corticosteroids, both inhaled and systemic, are used in the treatment of COPD and asthma. Systemic steroids produce a considerable number of physical side effects that are well known. Among these side effects is the possibility of an increase in anxiety, aggressiveness, and possibly psychosis [10]. Inhaled steroids produce far fewer side effects than systemic steroids.
- Theophylline is an oral bronchodilator of the methylxanthine class. In recent years theophylline has been used less in patients with lung disease because of its narrow therapeutic window and the effectiveness of other bronchodilator medications [5]. Theophylline is closely related to caffeine, another methylxanthine. The chemical structure of theophylline and caffeine differ by one methyl group. Theophylline may produce nausea, agitation, increased heart rate, tremor, and insomnia.

Heart Disease

Heart disease is a very common ailment in the United States. In general, heart disease may be divided into two categories: congenital and acquired. The following discussion centers predominately on acquired heart disease.

Coronary heart disease is the most common form of heart disease [11]. Cardiovascular diseases altogether are the leading cause of mortality in the United States [11]. Atherosclerosis of the coronary arteries is ultimately responsible for myocardial infarction, congestive heart failure, cardiac arrhythmia, and angina pectoris. These conditions, collectively, affect over 20 million adults. Symptoms of heart disease include the following [12]:

- Shortness of breath
- Chest pain
- Palpitations
- Syncope or presyncope
- Fatigue

Many of the symptoms of heart disease are not specific and may overlap with many other diseases. Heart disease symptoms are also closely similar to the symptoms of an anxiety disorder. The practitioner should also be aware that patients with heart disease may also suffer from a coexistent anxiety disorder.

Patients with congestive heart failure (CHF) may suffer from anxiety disorders (18%) and depression (29%) [13]. These disorders have been studied in CHF patients. Although anxiety is common in CHF patients, it is not associated with poor outcomes. On the other hand, depression in CHF patients has been associated with a worse prognosis [14]. Patients recently discharged from the hospital for CHF treatment have demonstrated higher levels of anxiety and depression [15]. The recognition of anxiety and depression in patients with heart disease and CHF is important and must be addressed.

Since the symptoms of heart disease and anxiety may overlap, it may be difficult for the practitioner to distinguish them. The following points may be helpful to the practitioner in the evaluation of patients with the common symptoms of both heart disease and anxiety:

- Palpitations: Palpitations are common patient complaints. Palpitations may be characterized as rapid or irregular heart beat, fluttering, or thumping sensations in the chest. Heart disease and anxiety are the two most common causes of palpitations [16]. When palpitations are associated with syncope, the likelihood of a serious cause is increased. Some medications and substances with stimulant properties may produce palpitations. Supraventricular and ventricular arrhythmias may occur with variable frequency [12]. Holter monitoring and event recording may be of great help in discovering the cause of palpitations. No etiology is discovered in 16% of patients with palpitations.
- Chest pain: Chest pain is a subjective term for the discomfort associated with acute coronary insufficiency. Chest pain may

come from a variety of causes including coronary heart disease and ventricular ischemia, pulmonary embolus, aortic dissection, costochondritis, esophagitis, gallbladder disease, pneumothorax, myocarditis, mitral valve prolapse, and pulmonary hypertension [12]. The chest pain symptom of acute coronary ischemia may occur as an isolated event, but is often associated with dyspnea, weakness, diaphoresis, and decreased ventricular output. Chest pain may also occur as a result of an anxiety disorder. The associated symptoms of decreased cardiac output are usually absent.

- Shortness of breath: Shortness of breath may occur frequently in patients with heart disease, especially in those affected by congestive heart failure. Patients with panic disorder may also experience shortness of breath as a result of hyperventilation. The dyspnea of CHF is usually worse when lying down and may be associated with jugular venous distention, hepatomegaly, peripheral edema, and cyanosis. The shortness of breath commonly seen in panic disorder is described as an inability to achieve a full, deep breath. There may also be a choking feeling as if something is lodged in the throat. Typically there is no cyanosis in panic disorder.

Physical examination may be beneficial in determining the difference between heart disease and an anxiety disorder. Patients with CHF may have rales on chest auscultation. The presence of wheezing or pleural effusion also supports the diagnosis of CHF. The presence of a third or fourth heart sound would indicate ventricular dysfunction.

While the above findings may help establish the diagnosis of CHF, the existence of an anxiety disorder is not necessarily discounted. However, the practitioner may prefer to address the CHF treatment with a greater priority.

The treatment of anxiety disorders in patients suffering from heart disease may include short-acting benzodiazepines, selective serotonin reuptake inhibitors (SSRIs), and tricyclic antidepressants (TCAs). Much has been written regarding the safety of SSRI and TCA medications in patients with coronary heart disease. Some reports indicate an increased risk to heart disease patients from the use of TCA or SSRI therapy [17]. Other studies indicate the relative safety of antidepressant therapy, especially the SSRI group [18]. Some research indicates the possibility of antiplatelet activity of SSRIs and a potential benefit from their use in coronary heart disease patients [19]. The practitioner may wish to consider the risk versus benefit of treatment with antidepressant medications in patients with heart disease. The patient who suffers from an anxiety disorder with coexistent heart disease carries a significant health burden. The practitioner must recognize this fact and consider offering medical therapy, when appropriate, for both illnesses.

Hyperthyroidism

Excessive production of thyroxine (thyrotoxicosis) produces the symptoms and physical findings of hyperthyroidism. There are multiple causes for this disorder; however, the most common cause is Graves' disease. Graves' disease is an autoimmune disorder affecting the thyroid gland that causes the increased production and release of thyroid hormone [20]. This disease is more common in women (8:1). Onset is usually between 20 and 40 years.

Symptoms of Graves' disease include nervousness, restlessness, heat intolerance, weakness, diarrhea, weight loss, palpitations, and menstrual irregularities [20]. Hyperthyroidism may be confused with an anxiety disorder or psychotic state, particularly mania. Hyperthyroidism onset is usually insidious. The anxiety symptoms may serve to delay diagnosis or cause initial misdiagnosis [21].

Use of an anxiety scale such as the Hamilton Anxiety Scale (HAS) [22] may be beneficial in differentiating the symptom profile in patients who initially present with either an anxiety disorder or hyperthyroidism [23]. The HAS employs questions that help define the anxiety symptoms in such a way to assist the practitioner in making a more definitive diagnosis.

Dietary Intake

Substances taken in the diet may produce stimulant-like effects. There are numerous substances that have been studied. The following is a discussion of two common dietary substances that may play a role in the evolution of anxiety symptoms:

- Caffeine: Caffeine is a methylxanthine compound that may produce tremor, alertness, nausea, nervousness, and anxiety, especially in large doses. It is one of the most widely used psychoactive substances worldwide [24]. Caffeine has been shown to produce anxiety symptoms in otherwise normal individuals and make anxiety-prone patients worse [24]. Psychosis may be induced by toxic doses of caffeine. The practitioner is wise to be aware of the potentially toxic effects of caffeine and should include caffeine intake as a part of the initial patient history.

- Monosodium glutamate: Monosodium glutamate (MSG) is a common substance used in food preparation as a flavor enhancer. Some patients may experience a stimulant-like effect following ingestion of MSG, which may be interpreted as an anxiety disorder. This has led to the coining of the term *Chinese restaurant syndrome* based on the belief that MSG is common to the preparation of Oriental cuisine. International study has concluded that a certain subgroup of the general population may be sensitive to MSG and experience restlessness, anxiety, and nervousness. The report also concluded that MSG is a safe compound and poses no unusual risk in general for human consumption [25]. The link to the Chinese restaurant syndrome was not established in this study.

Cancer

Perhaps no other condition can strike more fear, apprehension, and anxiety in a patient than the diagnosis of cancer. The anxiety that often surrounds the discussion of cancer poses a challenge not only for the patient but also for the practitioner. In late life, when cancer development is more likely, 20% of patients develop anxiety [26]. Despite this fact, very few studies have addressed the subject of anxiety in the older age group. There is literature, however, that discusses cognitive behavior therapy and other psychotherapeutic approaches to the patient with cancer. Psychotherapy has been used to reduce anxiety and other psychological symptoms in cancer patients [27]. Complex issues such as religious beliefs, family relationships, finances, and physical pain may face the patient who is dying of cancer. Many patients look to family members or clergy for help and support. The patient often regards the practitioner as a source of strength, comfort, and assistance. This is a role that the practitioner should not ignore. In terminally ill cases, the role of the practitioner turns from one of cure to one of comfort.

Providing education to patients about cancer risk, prevention, and treatment is a major role for many primary care practitioners. Considerable levels of anxiety that accompany the diagnosis of cancer may prevent the patient from understanding and comprehending the health care information that the practitioner may provide [28]. Since the patient's understanding of their illness is critical to the outcome of treatment, helping the patient deal with the anxiety about cancer may be as important as the cancer therapy itself. A calm and reassuring approach to the patient with cancer is the primary step in helping to allay the patient's anxiety. The use of benzodiazepine medications is proper and useful in most cases.

Alprazolam (Xanax) 0.5 to 1 mg twice a day or lorazepam (Ativan) 1 mg twice a day are two examples of benzodiazepines helpful in treating symptoms of anxiety.

Irritable Bowel Syndrome

Irritable bowel syndrome (IBS) is a common problem encountered by the primary care practitioner accounting for 3% of all patient visits [29]. Symptoms of abdominal pain, bloating, nausea, diarrhea, and constipation are commonly seen in these patients. Symptoms tend to be chronic in nature. The cause of irritable bowel syndrome is unknown. There is a theory that IBS is caused by a disorder of the brain–gut link mediated by corticotropin-releasing hormone [30]. Anxiety disorders and depression are commonly seen as comorbid conditions with irritable bowel syndrome [31].

Treatment of IBS is multidimensional. Alosetron (Lotronex), a 5-hydroxytryptamine-3 (5-HT3) antagonist, is approved for use in irritable bowel syndrome (32). There are precautions with its use and the practitioner is referred to the package prescribing information for more detail.

Selective serotonin reuptake inhibitors (SSRIs) are helpful in the treatment of IBS and the anxiety and depressive symptoms commonly associated with this disorder. Cognitive behavior therapy in conjunction with SSRI therapy has provided benefit to these patients as well [33].

A trial of sertraline (Zoloft), paroxetine (Paxil), fluoxetine (Prozac), citalopram (Celexa), or escitalopram (Lexapro) may be a helpful strategy in IBS patients. Venlafaxine (Effexor) and duloxetine (Cymbalta) may offer some benefit, but current studies are lacking. Table 13.1 lists some physical causes of anxiety symptoms.

TABLE 13.1. Physical causes of anxiety symptoms

Cardiovascular
Arrhythmia
Congestive heart failure
Coronary heart disease
Hypertension
Hypovolemia/hypoperfusion
Myocardial infarction
Valvular disease (congenital and acquired)

Continued

TABLE 13.1. *Continued*

Dietary
Caffeine
MSG
Vitamin deficiencies

Drug-related
Anticholinergic effect
Antihypertensives
Bronchodilators
Hallucinogens
Nicotine
Stimulants

Hematological
Anemia (B_{12} and iron-deficiency)

Rheumatological
Degenerative disk disease
Related inflammatory diseases
Systemic lupus erythematosus

Metabolic
Cushing's disease
Hyperthyroidism
Hypocalcemia
Hyponatremia
Hypothyroidism
Menopause

Neurological
Encephalopathies
Intracranial mass
Ménière syndrome
Seizure disorders (especially complex partial
   seizures)
Vertigo

Respiratory
Asthmatic bronchitis (intermittent and persistent)
Chronic obstructive pulmonary disease
Hemoptysis
Pneumonia
Pneumothorax
Pulmonary edema
Pulmonary embolism

Secreting tumors
Carcinoid syndrome
Pheochromocytoma

Adapted from ref. [34].

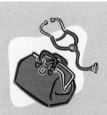

Pearls for the Practitioner

- Many patients with even a relatively minor medical problem may experience apprehension and anxiety associated with their illness. Primary care practitioners see a myriad of medical problems in the daily practice of medicine. The patient may be a fear that a symptom of an acute illness or change in symptoms of a chronic illness may signal the onset of a catastrophic event.

- Major emergencies in the daily practice of medicine are uncommon. The practitioner may be comfortable with the daily routine of a medical practice; however, the patient may not appreciate such insight and experience. Patients suffering from anxiety disorders often see their symptoms as signs of an impending medical calamity. Often the practitioner's calm reassurance alone will suffice to allay patient anxiety.

- The practitioner's recommendation for further x-rays, scans, lab work, and other tests may instill considerable anxiety in the patient. In the treatment of many medical conditions, the performance of diagnostic testing is often required. Explanation of the indications for testing and presentation of a reasonable expectation for the testing outcome may help to ease the tension and anxiety that accompanies undergoing "tests."

- The converse of the above may also occur. Some patients may be so apprehensive about their illness that they may desire or demand diagnostic testing. Often this desire stems from the patient's underlying anxiety state. Diagnostic testing may be perceived by some patients as being more specific and sensitive than is often the case. Recognition of this anxiety, addressing the apprehension, and informing the patient about diagnostic testing pros and cons may go a long way to improving patient comfort.

Continued

Continued

> • Many medications have a stimulant effect that may be inter-
> preted as anxiety. When a patient presents with a new com-
> plaint or symptom, it is wise for the practitioner to consider
> that the new symptom may be due to a medication side effect
> and not necessarily to the disease itself. Reducing dosage or
> changing medication often suffices to eliminate a stimulant
> side effect without losing the desired effect for its use.

References

1. Marciniak M, et al. The cost of treating anxiety: the medical and demo-
   graphic correlates that impact total medical costs. Depression and
   Anxiety 2005;21:178–184.
2. Dolnak D. Treating patients for comorbid depression, anxiety disorders, and somatic illness. JAOA 2006;106(5, suppl 2):S1–8.
3. First M, Frances A, Pincus H. Anxiety disorders. In: American
   Psychiatric Association. Diagnostic and Statistical Manual of Mental
   Disorders, 4th ed., text revision (DSM-IV-TR). Washington, DC: American
   Psychiatric Publishing, 2002:163–181.
4. Drooker M. Other cognitive disorders and mental disorders due to a
   general medical condition. In: Sadock B, Sadock V, eds. Comprehensive
   Textbook of Psychiatry. Philadelphia: Lippincott Williams & Wilkins,
   2005:1106–1136.
5. Chesnutt M, Prendergast T. Lung. In: Tierney L, McPhee S, Papadakis M,
   eds. Current Medical Diagnosis and Treatment. New York: McGraw-Hill,
   2006:218–311.
6. Roundy K, et al. Are anxiety and depression addressed in primary care
   patients with chronic obstructive pulmonary disease. J Clin Psychiatry
   Prim Care Companion 2005;7(5):213–217.
7. Hu J, Meek P. Health-related quality of life in individuals with chronic
   obstructive pulmonary disease. Heat Lung 2005;34(6):415–422.
8. Lavoie K, et al. Are psychiatric disorders associated with worse
   asthma control and quality of life in asthma patients? Respir Med
   2005;99:1249–1257.
9. Hoffman B, Lefkowitz R. Catecholamines and sympathomimetic
   drugs. In: Goodman A, Gilman A, Rall T, Nies A, Taylor P, eds. The
   Pharmacologic Basis of Therapeutics. Elmsford, NY: Pergamon Press,
   1990:187–220.
10. Kayani S, Shannon D. Adverse behavioral effects of treatment for
    acute exacerbations of asthma in children: a comparison of two doses
    of oral steroids. Chest 2002;122:624–628.
11. Thom T, et al. Heart disease and stroke statistics—2006 update.
    Circulation 2006;113:e85–e151.
12. Bashore T, Granger C. Heart. In: Tierney L, McPhee S, Papadakis M,
    eds. Current Medical Diagnosis and Treatment. New York: McGraw-
    Hill, 2006:312–418.

13. Haworth J, et al. Prevalence and predictors of anxiety and depression in a sample of chronic heart failure patients with left ventricular systolic dysfunction. Eur J Heart 2005;7(5):803–808.
14. Jaing W, et al. Prognostic value of anxiety and depression in patients with chronic heart failure. Circulation 2004;110(22):3452–3456.
15. Moser D, Doering L, Chung M. Vulnerabilities of patients recovering from an exacerbation of chronic heart failure. Am Heart J 2005;150(5):984.e7–13.
16. Abbott A. Diagnostic approach to palpitations. Am Fam Physician 2005;71(4):743–750.
17. Tata L, et al. General population based study of the impact of tri-cyclic and selective serotonin reuptake inhibitor antidepressants on the risk of acute myocardial infarction. Heart 2005;91:465–471.
18. Roose S, Miyazaki M. Pharmacologic treatment of depression in patients with heart disease. Psychosom Med 2005;67(S1):s54–57.
19. Schlienger R, Meier C. Effect of selective serotonin reuptake inhibitors on platelet activation: can they prevent acute myocardial infarction? Am J Cardiovasc Drugs 2003;3(3):149–162.
20. Fitzgerald P. Endocrinology. In: Current Medical Diagnosis and Treatment. New York: McGraw-Hill, 2006:1098–1193.
21. Stern R, et al. A survey study of neuropsychiatric complaints in patients with Graves' disease. J Neuropsychiatry Clin Neurosci 1996;8(2):181–185.
22. Sajatovic M, Ramirez L. Rating Scales in Mental Health. Hudson, OH: Lexi-Comp, 2003.
23. Iacovides A, et al. Difference in symptom profile between generalized anxiety disorder and anxiety secondary to hyperthyroidism. Int J Psychiatry Med 2000;30(1):71–81.
24. Broderick P, Benjamin A. Caffeine and psychiatric symptoms: a review. J Okla State Med Assoc 2004;97(12):538–542.
25. Walker R, Lupien J. The safety evaluation of monosodium glutamate. J Nutr 2000;130:1049s–1052s.
26. Ostir G, Goodwin J. High anxiety is associated with an increased risk if death in an older tri-ethnic population. J Clin Epidemiol 2006;59:534–540.
27. Cohen S, Block S. Issues in psychotherapy with terminally ill patients. Palliat Support Care 2004;2(2):181–189.
28. Stephenson P. Before the teaching begins: managing patient anxiety prior to providing education. Clin J Oncol Nurs 2006;10(2):241–245.
29. Spiller R. Irritable bowel syndrome. Br Med Bull 2005;72:15–29.
30. Sagami Y, et al. Effect of a corticotropin releasing hormone receptor antagonist on colonic sensory and motor function in patients with irritable bowel syndrome. Gut 2004;53(7):958–964.
31. Folks D. The interface of psychiatry and irritable bowel syndrome. Curr Psychiatry Rep 2004;6(3):210–215.
32. Haus U, Spath M, Farber L. Spectrum of use and tolerability of 5–HT3 receptor antagonists. Scand J Rheumatol Suppl 2004;119:12–18.
33. Jackson J, O'Malley P, Kroenke K. Antidepressants and cognitive behavioral therapy for symptom syndromes. CNS Spectrums 2006;11(3):212–222.
34. Chan P, Thomas D, McKinley E, Stanford E. Outpatient and Primary Care. Laguna Hills, CA: Current Clinical Strategies Publishing, 2005:232–255.

14

Anxiety Disorders
and Comorbidities

Lesa J. Feather, John K. Spraggins, and James D. Helsley

Diagnosing and managing anxiety disorders may be quite challenging at times. Time constraints and sheer patient volume may prohibit the primary care clinician from making complete and appropriate mental health diagnoses. It is not uncommon for a patient to have complex coexisting disorders with overlapping symptoms. Determining a primary versus a secondary diagnosis may also be difficult. Interestingly, long-term follow-up studies have shown that the development of an anxiety disorder is commonly followed by depression. With exceptions for the elderly, this sequence occurs more commonly than the development of depression followed by anxiety [1]. To increase practitioner awareness, this chapter reviews the comorbidities that may occur with anxiety disorders and offers general practical guidelines for therapy to improve global patient functioning. More in depth management strategies are discussed in the individual anxiety disorders chapters of this book.

HISTORY
The most crucial part of assessing the patient and accurately diagnosing an anxiety disorder is a complete history. A thorough patient history can often be obtained in a short period of time. Questionnaires or rating scales may be helpful assessment tools, and these can be self-administered or administered by trained staff. Reviewing information from the questionnaires with the patient helps to create good rapport as well. The practitioner must pay particular attention to crucial information such as bipolar symptoms, panic attacks, and suicidal behavior.

Common mental health adjunct assessment instruments include the Beck Anxiety Inventory (BAI), the Social Phobia Inventory (SPIN), the Florida Obsessive-Compulsive Inventory Screening Test (FOCI), the Beck Depression Inventory (BDI), the Mood Disorder Questionnaire (MDQ), and the Adult Self-Report Scale (ASRS) symptom checklist for adult attention-deficit hyperactivity disorder (ADHD). These instruments may also be used to help gauge remission/ recovery status during the course of treatment.

The Psychiatric Diagnostic Screening Questionnaire (PDSQ), a 126-question assessment, covers 13 *Diagnostic and Statistical Manual of Mental Disorders*, 4th edition (DSM-IV) disorders in five areas: eating, mood, anxiety, substance use, and somatoform disorders. The PDSQ assesses six specific DSM-IV anxiety disorders: panic disorder, agoraphobia, posttraumatic stress disorder (PTSD), obsessive-compulsive disorder (OCD), generalized anxiety disorder (GAD), and social phobia (social anxiety disorder). This instrument has been shown to have a high sensitivity and a high negative predictive value. The clinician may be confident when the screening test indicates that a disorder is not present [2].

ANXIETY DISORDERS WITH COMORBID DEPRESSION
There has been much debate regarding proper diagnostic classification for those individuals presenting with coexisting anxiety and depressive symptoms. In the first and second editions of the DSM, anxiety disorders and major depression were thought to be more alike than different. In the third edition in 1980, the DSM delineated exclusive classifications for anxiety and depressive disorders. In the late 1980s and early 1990s, yet another change ensued, establishing that a patient may develop an anxiety disorder and depression jointly. The DSM-III-R (1987) and DSM-IV (1994) allowed for the diagnosis of single disorders or multiple disorders concurrently [3].

Clinicians and researchers have also considered that depression and anxiety are not two separate coexisting disorders but rather two versions of the same disorder. Marano quotes David Barlow, PhD, director of the Center for Anxiety and Related Disorders at Boston University, states, "They're probably two sides of the same coin." He goes on to explain, "The genetics seem to be the same. The neurobiology seems to overlap. The psychological and biological nature of the vulnerability is the same. It just seems that some people with the vulnerability react with anxiety to life stressors. And some people, in addition, go beyond that to become depressed." He simplifies this by stating, "Anxiety is a kind of looking to the future, seeing dangerous things that might happen in the next hour, day or weeks. Depression is all that with the addition of 'I really don't think I'm going to be able to cope with this, maybe I'll just give up.' It's shut-down marked by mental, cognitive, or behavioral slowing" [4].

Practitioners still ponder which disorder comes first, anxiety or depression, only hoping to intervene before the second disorder ensues. Evidence shows that in two thirds of cases, early onset of anxiety disorders (generalized anxiety disorder [GAD], social anxiety disorder [SAD], posttraumatic stress disorder [PTSD]) predisposes to later onset of major depressive disorder (MDD) [5]. Interestingly, when dealing with panic disorder and coexisting MDD, the anxiety disorder only precedes the depression in one third of the cases [5]. The order of onset has not been shown to alter treatment outcomes, but is important for provider and patient awareness [5].

Patients who present with clinical depressive symptoms and are subsequently diagnosed with MDD may suffer from an anxiety disorder as well. Comorbid anxiety symptoms from the spectrum of anxiety disorders tend to make major depression more severe and prolonged, less likely to respond to treatment, and more functionally impairing in work activities, social accomplishments, and family roles [2]. More than 80% of depressed patients with comorbid anxiety continue to be depressed after 1 year, compared with less than 60% who have depression alone [2]. Patients with both depression and anxiety symptoms tend to be more prone to suicidality. These patients are likely to have a past history of suicide attempts, which may predict future thoughts or attempts [2].

When patients present primarily with anxiety symptoms, an anxiety disorder is often viewed as the primary disorder. The clinician may fail to recognize an underlying depression or other disorder that may be "driving" the anxiety symptoms. It has been documented by the National Comorbidity Survey (NCS) that 90% of those with lifetime GAD had other lifetime psychiatric diagnoses, most commonly major depression, dysthymia, substance abuse, simple phobia, and social phobia [1]. Studies invariably report higher comorbidity with GAD than with other anxiety disorders [1]. In prospective studies, patients with anxious symptoms are more likely to develop major depression on exposure to stressful life events. After remission of depression, GAD symptoms may remain [1].

RISK FACTORS FOR ANXIETY DISORDERS AND DEPRESSION

Risk factors for developing both anxiety disorders and depression include the following [4]:

- Family history: Anxiety disorders and depression tend to occur from generation to generation.
- Type of anxiety disorder: Obsessive-compulsive disorder (OCD), panic disorder, and social phobia are particularly associated with depression. Specific phobias are associated less often.

- Age: Patients who develop an anxiety disorder for the first time after age 40 are more likely to suffer from depression. The average age of the first onset of an anxiety disorder is the mid-20s [4].

TREATMENT OF ANXIETY DISORDERS AND DEPRESSION

The presence of depression and a comorbid anxiety disorder, particularly panic disorder and GAD, may influence the antidepressant selected [2]. Pharmacotherapy for anxiety disorders with comorbid major depression includes antidepressants, benzodiazepines, and other agents such as buspirone (BuSpar). Antidepressants that may be helpful for comorbid anxiety disorders and depression include selective serotonin reuptake inhibitors (SSRIs), serotonin-norepinephrine reuptake inhibitors (SNRIs), mirtazapine (Remeron), tricyclic antidepressants (TCAs), and the monamine oxidase inhibitors (MAOIs).

Before prescribing an antidepressant, it is important to rule out a family or personal history of bipolar disorder. Initiation of antidepressant therapy alone in a patient with bipolar depression could induce a hypomanic or manic phase. It is particularly important to inquire about a family history of substance abuse, suicidal behavior, past hospitalizations, and failed treatment regimens. This may help determine the patient's risk for bipolar disorder. Utilization of a screening questionnaire such as the Mood Disorder Questionnaire (MDQ) can be helpful.

Benzodiazepines may be prescribed as monotherapy or as adjunctive treatment for many anxiety disorders. Benzodiazepines, when used cautiously and appropriately, may be very effective for the anxiety symptoms. If used long-term, the patient may develop physical dependence and experience withdrawal upon discontinuation. Benzodiazepines may also worsen a comorbid depression.

The SSRIs and SNRIs are recommended as first-line medications in the treatment of anxiety and depressive disorders because they are very efficacious and relatively safe. These medications may be associated with some initial energizing effects that can make patients with anxiety disorders more anxious and jittery. For this reason, therapy should be started at the lowest doses and titrated upward slowly. Adding a benzodiazepine for short-term use initially may counter some of the energizing effects. For example, adding a benzodiazepine to an antidepressant may be helpful during the initial 3 to 6 weeks of treatment until the SSRIs or SNRIs become therapeutic. The benzodiazepine may then be tapered and discontinued.

Buspirone (BuSpar) is a nonbenzodiazepine anxiolytic lacking sedative effects. It is indicated for the treatment of GAD. It may occasionally be clinically useful as an adjunct to an antidepressant such as an SSRI. For short-term management of anxiety symptoms, the antihistamine hydroxyzine pamoate (Vistaril) may be helpful, especially when sedative effects are desired. Further information on the treatment of anxiety disorders is discussed in the individual chapters of this book.

TREATMENT OF ANXIETY DISORDERS WITH COMORBID DEPRESSION
Examples of treatment for specific anxiety disorders with comorbid depression include the following:

- Obsessive-compulsive disorder (OCD) with major depression: The SSRIs approved by the U.S. Food and Drug Administration (FDA) for the treatment of OCD include fluoxetine (Prozac), fluvoxamine (Luvox), sertraline (Zoloft), and paroxetine (Paxil). Antidepressants used in conjunction with cognitive behavior therapy (CBT) may be very helpful in the treatment of comorbid OCD and depression.
- Generalized anxiety disorder with major depression: The SSRIs escitalopram (Lexapro) and paroxetine (Paxil) are FDA approved for GAD and MDD. The SNRIs venlafaxine extended release (Effexor XR) and duloxetine (Cymbalta) are indicated for both GAD and MDD. Cognitive behavior therapy has proven beneficial for patients with both GAD and depression.
- Panic disorder with major depression: The SSRIs approved by the FDA for the treatment of panic disorder include fluoxetine (Prozac), paroxetine (Paxil, Paxil CR), and sertraline (Zoloft). The key to starting an SSRI regimen in panic disorder is to "start low and go slow." Initial excitation from SSRIs may worsen symptoms of panic disorder. The initiation of a short-acting benzodiazepine may be helpful. Patients need to be reassured that the medications will help decrease anxiety symptoms in the long term. Cognitive behavior therapy is also useful, including muscle relaxation and breathing retraining. Psychoeducation enables patients to better understand their disorder. Cognitive behavior therapy for panic disorder has proven effective in the presence of depression.
- Social phobia (social anxiety disorder) with major depression: Social anxiety disorder and depression may coexist. The SSRIs are recommended as first-line pharmacotherapy. The SSRIs approved by the FDA for the treatment of social anxiety disorder include paroxetine (Paxil, Paxil CR) and sertraline (Zoloft), but response has been shown with many of the other SSRIs.

- Posttraumatic stress disorder (PTSD) with major depression: High rates of depression may occur during the course of PTSD [3]. Previously diagnosed depression is a risk factor for developing PTSD following exposure to a traumatic event [3]. The SSRIs with an FDA-approved indication for PTSD include paroxetine (Paxil) and sertraline (Zoloft). Psychotherapy involving repeated imagined exposure to traumatic memories and in vivo exposure to situations is often beneficial in the treatment of PTSD [3].

ANXIETY DISORDERS AND COMORBID BIPOLAR DISORDER

Determining the presence of bipolar disorder is of utmost importance in the clinical evaluation. If the diagnosis of bipolar disorder is considered, it is wise to initially direct treatment toward that disorder. Bipolar disorder, especially bipolar depression, is frequently not recognized and therefore may go undiagnosed, even by expert clinicians. A general understanding of bipolar disorders is important, and the primary care practitioner must consider bipolar disorder in all patients with anxiety and mood disorders. Although a patient's primary symptoms may appear to indicate a straightforward anxiety disorder diagnosis such as panic disorder, it is important to rule out a mood disorder. Certain clues in the history may signal further inquiry such as a history of suicidal behavior, multiple failed medication regimens, substance abuse, school or occupational failure, multiple failed marriages, and episodic antisocial behaviors [6]. Mood disorder questionnaires may help establish the diagnosis of bipolar disorder and may prompt further discussion. Other psychiatric disorders may mimic the symptoms of a bipolar disorder, so differentiating them may require a more extensive evaluation.

Bipolar disorder is diagnosed as type I, type II, or cyclothymia. Bipolar I disorder is characterized by one or more occurrences of mania. The essential feature of bipolar II disorder is the presence of one or more major depressive episodes accompanied by at least one hypomanic episode. Cyclothymic disorder is diagnosed in the presence of numerous hypomanic episodes that do not meet the criteria for manic episodes and numerous bouts of depression that do not meet the criteria for a major depressive episode.

Bipolar disorder generally develops during adolescence or young adulthood. If a hypomanic episode occurs after the age of 40 years, a general medical condition should be suspected. Hypomanic episodes occur more frequently in men than do major depressive episodes, and for women the reverse holds true [6]. Women are more prone to rapid cycling. Evidence also suggests that mixed or depressive symptoms during hypomania are more common in women [6]. Subsequent mood episodes may occur in the postpartum period or in the premenstrual phase [6]. There is evidence of a strong genetic influence. Individuals with a first-degree biological relative with bipolar disorder have increased rates of occurrence [6].

MOOD STABILIZATION

If a patient presents with severe anxiety symptoms and has a diagnosis of bipolar disorder, caution should be taken when pre-scribing adjunctive therapy. Once mood stabilization has been achieved, the practitioner may cautiously proceed with adding other medications to treat the anxiety disorder [7]. The clinician must be very careful when using antidepressants in a patient who has bipolar disorder, closely monitoring for hypomanic or manic symptoms. Paroxetine (Paxil, Paxil CR) has shown the least risk of inducing mania, whereas venlafaxine (Effexor, Effexor XR) may be the most likely to induce mania [8]. Patient education is para-mount for successful management.

ANXIETY DISORDERS AND COMORBID ADULT ATTENTION-DEFICIT HYPERACTIVITY DISORDER

Determining the presence of either anxiety or adult attention-deficit hyperactivity disorder (ADHD) can be a challenge to the primary care practitioner. Some primary care providers may not feel experienced enough to diagnose and treat adult ADHD, and some psychiatric specialists are uncomfortable with the treatment of ADHD as well [7]. By definition, patients with ADHD must have presenting symptoms before the age of 7 years, but it may be many years later before ADHD is recognized and a diagnosis is made.

Individuals with ADHD tend to make careless mistakes with schoolwork or on the job, often appear as if they are not listening, cannot maintain attention for sustained periods of time, and often jump from one incomplete task to another. Work habits may be disorganized and materials are often scattered or misplaced. Minor distractions can pull an individual away from current tasks.

Hyperactivity in adults often presents as extreme fidgetiness or squirminess, such as shaking the feet or bouncing the legs. Impulsivity manifests as difficulty waiting one's turn in line, inter-rupting others, and blurting out information or answers at inap-propriate times.

Attention-deficit hyperactivity disorder symptoms initially present in the elementary school years, whereas anxiety disorders tend to present in late adolescence to the early 20s. Children may also suffer from various anxiety disorders, particularly separation anxiety disorder, social phobia, and obsessive-compulsive disorder [4]. Age is certainly a factor to consider when making the diagnosis of an anxiety disorder [4]. Anxiety disorders can also cause poor concentration, sleep problems, and difficulty with social, academic, and occupational functioning. Difficulty sleeping and excessive worry may occur secondary to ADHD because of apprehension and worry about deadlines and performance. Anxiety disorders may need to be treated successfully prior to treating symptoms of ADHD. Pharmacotherapy for ADHD can worsen anxiety symptoms in some patients, especially when dealing with panic-related anxiety. The practitioner must recognize, however, that anxiety symptoms stemming from untreated ADHD may be a significant clinical issue that requires treatment sooner rather than later.

The Adult Self-Report Scale Symptom Checklist (ASRS) for ADHD is a very useful and quick screening device for adult patients. Questionnaire results and clinical history can help the practitioner determine the primary diagnosis. It is not unusual for ADHD symptoms to present as a primary diagnosis with secondary anxiety symptoms.

There are several medications available on the market today to treat adult ADHD. The FDA-approved medications for the treatment of adult ADHD include amphetamine salt combination extended release (Adderall XR) and dexmethylphenidate extended release (Focalin XR), as well as the nonstimulant atomoxetine (Strattera). The cautious treatment of adult ADHD in the presence of currently treated comorbid psychiatric disorders such as the anxiety disorders is an important aspect of comprehensive patient management.

ANXIETY DISORDERS AND COMORBID PERSONALITY DISORDERS

The *Diagnostic and Statistical Manual of Mental Disorders,* 4th edition, text revision (DSM-IV-TR) defines a personality disorder as "an enduring pattern of inner experience and behavior that deviates markedly from the expectations of the individual's culture, is pervasive and inflexible, has an onset in adolescence or early adulthood, is stable over time, and leads to distress or impairment." The DSM-IV-TR classifies 10 personality disorders into three clusters (6):

- Cluster A: The "eccentric" cluster consists of paranoid personality disorder, schizoid personality disorder and schizotypal personality disorder.

- Cluster B: The "dramatic" cluster consists of antisocial personality disorder, borderline personality disorder, histrionic personality disorder and narcissistic personality disorders.
- Cluster C: The "anxious" cluster consists of avoidant personality disorder, dependent personality disorder and obsessive-compulsive personality disorder.

DEFINITIONS OF EACH PERSONALITY DISORDER AS LISTED IN THE DSM-IV-TR

Paranoid: a pattern of distrust and suspiciousness such that others' motives are interpreted as malevolent.

Schizoid: a pattern of detachment from social relationships and a restricted range of emotional expression.

Schizotypal: a pattern of acute discomfort in close relationships, cognitive or perceptual distortions, and eccentricities of behavior.

Antisocial: a pattern of disregard for, and violation of, the rights of others.

Borderline: a pattern of instability in interpersonal relationships, self-image, and affects, and marked impulsivity.

Histrionic: a pattern of excessive emotionality and attention seeking.

Narcissistic: a pattern of grandiosity, need for admiration, and lack of empathy.

Avoidant: a pattern of social inhibition, feelings of inadequacy, and hypersensitivity to negative evaluation.

Dependent: a pattern of submissive and clinging behavior related to an excessive need to be taken care of.

Obsessive-compulsive: a pattern of preoccupation with orderliness, perfectionism, and control.

Personality disorder not otherwise specified (NOS): for patients that fulfill criteria from each category, but do not meet criteria for one single personality disorder [6].

Many patients with anxiety disorders have a personality disorder [9]. The most common personality disorders encountered in patients with anxiety disorders are avoidant and dependent personality disorders. Social phobia is more commonly associated with a personality disorder than any other anxiety disorder [9]. Anxiety disorders tend to be more severe in patients with a comorbid personality disorder. [9].

Personality characteristics must take into account the patient's ethnic, cultural, and social background [6]. For example, problems associated with immigrants trying to adapt to a new culture should not be confused with personality disorders. Loss of an emotional support system and drastic changes in environment (e.g., death of a spouse, loss of a job) can exacerbate the symptoms of a personality disorder. Personality traits may be diagnosed as a personality disorder only when they are, "inflexible, maladaptive, and persisting and cause significant functional impairment or subjective distress" [6].

ANXIETY DISORDERS AND COMORBID SUBSTANCE ABUSE

The coexistence of a substance abuse disorder must always be considered when treating an anxiety disorder. Recent studies have shown that the prevalence of dual-diagnosed patients has increased. Research indicates that it is quite common for addiction to involve multiple drugs. Simultaneous treatment of other mental disorders has become the status quo, whereas in the past, it was thought that substance abuse difficulties needed to be addressed prior to the treatment of other mental health issues [10].

Identifying substance abuse may be a difficult task for the primary care practitioner. Patient denial is a part of the addiction process. Underreporting of substance use is an aspect of denial. Because clinical interviews are time-limited, collaboration is always helpful [11].

It has been observed that patients who abuse substances often become addicted to alcohol first. Most alcohol abusers under the age of 30 years are actually polysubstance abusers [10]. Approximately 9% of the U.S. adult population has a mood disorder. Estimates are that >9% of mood disorder patients abuse substances [10].

Individuals may abuse or become addicted to alcohol or other substances (e.g., marijuana, benzodiazepines) because of the anxiety reducing qualities of the drugs. Anxiety and stress exacerbate many other conditions [12].

There appears to be a strong relationship between teenage substance abuse and adult abuse/addiction [13]. Research has shown that the treatment of patients with substance abuse may be complicated by a multitude of psychological, behavioral, and physical factors resulting from early substance exposure [14].

The primary care practitioner must be aware of the possibility of substance abuse in patients with anxiety disorders. Regular screening is very important. It is sometimes clinically difficult to determine whether the patient abuses substance to "self-medicate" an anxiety disorder, whether the substance use causes anxiety symptoms, or both. According to Mersy [15], at least 20% of patients have some type of substance abuse issue. The primary care practitioner serves an important role in the identification, treatment, and referral process.

References

1. Stein D. Comorbidity in generalized anxiety disorder: impact and implications. J Clin Psychiatry 2001;62(11):29–34.
2. Thase M, Fave M, Zimmerman M, Culpeper L. Review of pharmacologic management of depression. J Clin Psychiatry Prim Care Companion 2006;8(2):88–97.
3. Rosenbaum J, Fredman S. Treatment of anxiety disorders with comorbid depression. Medscape from WEB MD June 2002. www.medscape.com.
4. Marano H. Anxiety and depression together. Psych Today 2003:1–2 (October).
5. Simon N, Rosenbaum J. Anxiety and depression comorbidity: implications and intervention. Medscape Psychiatry and Mental Health 2003;8(1):1–4. www.medscape.com.
6. American Psychiatric Association. Diagnostic and Statistical Manual of Mental Disorders, 4th ed., text revision. Washington, DC: American Psychiatric Association, 2000.
7. Arana G, Hyman S, Rosenbaum J, ed. Handbook of Psychiatric Drug Therapy, 4th ed. Philadelphia: Lippincott Williams & Wilkins, 2001:114–169, 210–236.
8. Masand P, ed., Rapaport M, Thase M. New direction for improved treatment of unipolar and bipolar depression. Psych CME Classic 2005:1(11):1–6.
9. VanVelzen C, Emmelkamp P. The relationship between anxiety disorders and personality disorders: prevalence rates and comorbidity models. In: Derksen J, Maffei C, Groen H, eds. Treatment of Personality Disorders. New York: Kluwer Academic/Plenum Publishers, 1999:129–153.
10. Miller N. Relationship of psychiatric and addictive disorders: an overview. In: Miller NS, ed. Addiction Psychiatry: Current diagnosis and Treatment. New York: Wiley and Sons, 1995:33–139.
11. Hitt M. More than 1 in 4 adults per year affected by mental illness or substance abuse. WEB MD June 2005. www.webmd.com.
12. Symptoms of anxiety. WEB MD October 2004. www.webmd.com.
13. Barlow D. Clinical Handbook of Psychological Disorders: A Step-by-Step Treatment Manual: Clinical Stress Management. New York, NY: Rosenthal and Rosenthal 1985:145–205.
14. Brems C, Johnson M, et al. Childhood abuse history and substance use among men and women receiving detoxification services. Am J Drug Alcohol Abuse 2004;30(4):799–821.
15. Mersy D. Anxiety disorders and substance abuse. Am Fam Phys 2003;67(7): 1529–1532.

15
Geriatric Anxiety and Anxiety Disorders

James D. Helsley and Sandra K. Vanin

In 1965, the federal government passed the Older Americans Act (OAA) and the Administration on Aging (AoA) was created. By that act, older Americans were considered to be persons 60 years of age or older. There are many terms used to define this population of individuals, including geriatric, senior, seasoned, and aged. This chapter uses these terms interchangeably. From a medical standpoint, age ranges vary when defining this population. As of 2004, there were 36.3 million people in the United States over the age of 65 years [1]. One in every eight Americans is an older citizen. Elderly women outnumber men by six million. The over-65 population in the United States is expected to reach 55 million by the year 2020. Approximately one third of the elderly live alone. Median income for the elderly in 2004 was $21,102 for males and $12,080 for females. One third of older Americans rely on Social Security for 90% of their income [1]. The average geriatric patient takes 3.2 drugs. Forty percent of the elderly take more than three drugs [1]. The most commonly consumed medications by patients over 65 years of age are listed in Table 15.1 [1].

The elderly are not immune to the development of anxiety symptoms and anxiety disorders. Primary care practitioners frequently encounter geriatric patients who present with anxiety symptoms and anxiety disorders. Many elderly live alone and worry about finances, personal safety, and independence. Many are widowed with no children living nearby. The anxiety disorders such as, generalized anxiety disorder (GAD), panic disorder, posttraumatic stress disorder (PTSD), obsessive-compulsive disorder (OCD), and phobias can all occur with advanced age. As with many other illnesses in the elderly, the symptoms of anxiety may not be distinct. The presentation of anxiety disorders may be clouded by coexisting medical or psychiatric illnesses, prior life experiences, medication side effects, and the changes in sensory, motor, and physiological function associated with aging.

TABLE 15.1. Commonly prescribed medications for the geriatric population

Antiarthritics	Beta-blockers
Thiazide diuretics	Digoxin
Potassium sparing diuretics	Loop diuretics
Nitrates	Antihypertensives (all others)
Diabetic oral agents	Benzodiazepines

Adapted from ref. [1].

Not all anxiety in the elderly mandates medical treatment intervention. For instance, some patients are fearful of ambulation because of a fear of falling or an anticipation of experiencing pain arising from joint disease [2]. In some patients, this may represent a legitimate fear and not simply apprehension without basis. Previous injury, pain with activity, or some prior untoward event may resurrect unpleasant memories that serve to keep the patient from activity. A few minutes spent by the practitioner simply listening to the patient can provide invaluable assistance in the care of the aged, not only with psychiatric issues but with general medical care as well.

Anxiety disorders occur more frequently in patients with chronic medical problems [2], and chronic medical problems are more common in the elderly. The increased impact on cost and usage of medical care services by patients with anxiety disorders, including panic, has been established [3]. Higher mortality rates have been observed in patients with anxiety disorders [2]. The proper diagnosis and treatment of anxiety disorders in the elderly is vital [4]. Little is written specifically about anxiety disorders in the elderly, yet anxiety symptoms are encountered frequently in geriatric medical practice. Causes of anxiety symptoms are varied. Common examples of illnesses that cause anxiety symptoms in older individuals are listed in Table 15.2 [5].

PHARMACOKINETICS AND AGING

Pharmacokinetics is defined as the study of drug absorption, metabolism, distribution, and elimination [6]. Throughout the human life span, anatomical and physiological changes occur that have great impact on pharmacokinetics. The understanding of illness and the medical therapy of elderly patients are tightly woven together with the relationship to drug pharmacokinetics. It is imperative for the practitioner who treats geriatric patients to have a working knowledge of these changes. The impact on medical therapy is great.

TABLE 15.2. Common examples of causes of anxiety symptoms in the older population

- General medical illness
  - Heart disease
  - Lung disease
  - Gastrointestinal (GI) diseases
  - Anemia
  - Metabolic disorders
  - Endocrine disorders
- Psychiatric illness
  - Major depression
  - Generalized anxiety disorders
  - Grief/mourning
  - Adjustment disorders
- Neurological disorders
  - Dementias
  - Delirium
  - Seizure disorders
  - Encephalopathies
  - Postconcussion syndrome
- Drugs/medications
  - Caffeine
  - Alcohol
  - Bronchodilators
  - Neuroleptics
  - Antihypertensives
  - Steroids
  - Diuretics
  - Anticholinergics
  - Hallucinogens
  - Stimulants

Adapted from ref. [5].

In order for a drug to be effective, it must first be absorbed. Several factors affect drug absorption in the elderly (Table 15.3) [6].

With advanced age, there is a shift toward less lean body mass. Relatively speaking, there is more adipose tissue (fat) and less muscle (lean body mass) in the elderly. This occurs even if there is no overall change in body weight. Water-soluble (hydrophilic) medications disperse throughout lean body mass as opposed to fat. Since lean body mass is less, the peak concentration of the more water-soluble medications is higher [6]. An example of a water-soluble medication is acetaminophen (Tylenol).

Lipophilic (fat-soluble) drugs behave differently. Fat-soluble drugs disperse and equilibrate throughout body fat stores and

TABLE 15.3. Factors affecting drug effectiveness in geriatric patients

- Decreased gastric acid production allowing for a higher gastric pH. Some medications are affected gastric pH and may dissolve and absorb more quickly or slowly.
- Geriatric patients have decreased splanchnic blood flow, which may result in less drug being absorbed.
- Decreased gastrointestinal motility is common with advanced age. This may affect medications that require entry into the small bowel to achieve absorption.
- The intestinal epithelium is generally less effective with advanced age. This may cause a lesser degree of drug absorption allowing more of the dose to remain in the gut.

Adapted from ref. [6].

tissues. As a result, peak serum concentrations are lower, but duration of action is longer. It takes more time for lipophilic drugs to diffuse from fat stores back into the serum for degradation and elimination. As a general rule, most psychoactive drugs are lipophilic and cross the blood–brain barrier, which is the dense lipid membrane of the cerebral vasculature. Hydrophilic drugs do not penetrate these membranes well [6].

While serum creatinine may remain within the laboratory normal range, it should be remembered that creatinine clearance diminishes with age. Even in the absence of known renal diseases, the creatinine clearance of a patient 80 years old is about half of that of a patient 25 years of age [6,7]. Since lean body mass declines with age, the production of creatinine and blood urea nitrogen also decline [6,7]. The net effect is a laboratory normal creatinine, despite the fact that creatinine clearance is dramatically reduced. Drugs that are excreted through renal mechanisms require lowered doses and close clinical monitoring for side effects. Examples of drugs excreted by the renal route include digoxin, aminoglycosides, lithium, gabapentin, and penicillin.

Many drugs are metabolized by the liver. Some must be first metabolized into an active form before the drug effect occurs. Hepatic phase 1 metabolism includes the processes of oxidation, reduction, and hydrolysis. These mechanisms decline with age. Many metabolites are as effective or more effective than the parent drug. These metabolites are generally more water-soluble than the parent compound. Phase 2 metabolism involves the conjugation to inactive metabolites. This process does not decline with age. In many cases, the change in hepatic drug metabolism means that decreased "first-pass" effect may yield more parent drug into the system. If the parent drug is the active compound, greater drug effect would be expected. If the parent drug requires metabolism to an active form, then a less immediate effect of the drug may be expected.

With age there is also a decrease in serum albumin. This decrease is much greater in geriatric patients who are ill, frail, or poorly nourished. Highly protein-bound (bound to albumin) medications may be available in the serum as free drugs and, hence, are likely to produce an effect or induce side effects.

DIFFERENTIAL DIAGNOSES IN GERIATRIC ANXIETY

Anxiety disorders in the elderly are usually not encountered as isolated diagnoses. Comorbidity tends to be more the rule than the exception. The following is a discussion of three common conditions that may affect behavior and play a significant role when associated with anxiety in the evaluation and treatment of geriatric patients.

Depression in the Elderly

Depression is a common ailment of the elderly population and may occur in as many as 50% or more of patients [3]. The symptoms of depression in the elderly may not be as obvious to the practitioner as the symptoms that occur in a younger patient [7,8]. Many elderly patients do not openly complain of being depressed or sad, but may complain of somatic physical symptoms that are not supported by a physical disorder. According to the *Diagnostic and Statistical Manual of Mental Disorders,* 4th edition, text revision (DSM-IV-TR), at least four symptoms from Table 15.4 must be present to make a diagnosis of major depression.

TABLE 15.4. Major depression in the geriatric patient: symptoms

At least four of the following symptoms must be present to make a diagnosis:

- Weight loss/gain, poor appetite
- Insomnia or excessive sleeping
- Psychomotor agitation or retardation
- Loss of interest, energy, enthusiasm
- Feelings of worthlessness, excessive guilt
- Decreased ability to concentrate or process thoughts
- Persistent, recurrent thought of death, suicide, suicide attempt, expression of wishes to be dead or "get it over with"

Adapted from *Diagnostic and Statistical Manual of Mental Disorders,* 4th edition, text revision (DSM-IV-TR).

Recognition of depression by the practitioner requires attention to the patient's demeanor, affect, and complaints. Often the clue to the correct diagnosis of depression is a subtle remark or gesture disguised in the presentation of the patient's initial complaint [7,8].

The grief reaction (bereavement) is a normal event following the loss of a loved one. Many elderly patients will lose a spouse or companion. Sadness, crying, anorexia, and even guilt feelings are common following a significant loss [7,9]. These emotions are normal and expected. Prolonged grieving may signal the diagnosis of depression. The definition of prolonged grieving is difficult to describe, as different cultures have different accepted grieving behaviors. In general, a period of 6 months or longer of sadness and symptoms of depression following a significant loss may be grounds for the practitioner to approach the patient about the possibility of depressive illness.

Depression in the elderly is associated with a higher rate of usage of medical services, increased consultation with specialists, increased need for assistance with activities of daily living (ADL), and a higher use of medication [4]. The implications are quite significant. Unrecognized and untreated depression in the elderly can lead to a decrease in the patient's sense of well-being and an increased use of health care services. Not all elderly patients with depression are withdrawn, sedate, sad, and tearful. Some patients experience psychomotor agitation as part of their depressive illness. This agitation may be interpreted as an anxiety disorder. While anxiety disorders do occur in the elderly [9,10], anxiety-like symptoms such as restlessness, agitation, and irritability may also occur in depressed elderly patients. Anxiety disorders and depression frequently coexist [11]. It is wise for the practitioner to be alert to the multiple array of symptoms with which the elderly patient may present, and work with the patient to achieve a correct diagnosis and plan for treatment.

Dementia

Some memory loss occurs as a normal process of aging [12]. Dementia is characterized as a precipitous decline in memory and recall, particularly of recent events. Memory loss in dementia progresses to the point where judgment becomes impaired. Some patients with dementia also develop behavioral disorders [13]. A wide range of behavioral symptoms may occur in elderly patients with dementia (Table 15.5).

Differentiating the symptoms of an emotional disorder from the symptoms of dementia poses a great challenge to the practitioner.

TABLE 15.5. Behavioral symptoms of dementia in the geriatric patient

- Psychotic features
  - Hallucinations
  - Delusions
  - Delusional misidentifications
- Nonpsychotic features
  - Agitation
  - Wandering
  - Aggression

Adapted from ref. [13].

Depression may give the appearance of dementia. The term *pseudodementia* was introduced by Wells [14] in 1979 to describe the unanticipated recovery of a patient who had the diagnosis of dementia. The consensus is that depression in the elderly can express itself as symptoms of dementia. Treatment for the depressive illness can lead to an improvement in the very symptoms that resembled those seen in dementia. Usually, a patient with dementia presents with symptoms of decline that occur in a gradual and progressive manner. Patients with pseudodementia may have a more abrupt onset of decreased cognitive function. Some patients with pseudodementia may have a remote history of depressive illness or other emotional disorder [7]. A detailed history is imperative in order for the practitioner to determine the onset of symptoms and their timeline. Frequently, this is a difficult task for the practitioner.

The Mini–Mental State Examination (MMSE) is an invaluable tool in the diagnostic workup of elderly patients with emotional, cognitive, and behavioral problems. Folstein et al. [15] in 1975 developed this questionnaire to help in the diagnosis of dementia in the elderly. It is a rather simple test to administer and can be performed by a trained member of the office staff.

Over the spectrum of dementias, anxiety plays a role in the diagnosis and therapy of elderly patients. In many patients, the mere presence of cognitive decline, whether natural or as a result of disease, can cause apprehension [4,10]. Anxiety symptoms associated with dementia may be the reason the elderly patient seeks care. Insomnia or other sleep problems, fear of falling, fear of pain, financial problems, and many other serious concerns may induce an anxiety state that the elderly patient may or may not understand [2,8].

Delirium

Many elderly patients experience acute confusional states [16]. A deterioration of clear cognition can be associated with and attributed to numerous causes (Table 15.6).

Symptoms of decreased alertness, slurred speech, agitation, disorientation, decreased attention, anxiety, and hallucinations are all common with delirium [17]. Symptoms of delirium and confusion can mimic some of the symptoms of a generalized anxiety state or panic disorder. It is important to attempt to differentiate the symptoms carefully in order to discover an underlying cause.

TABLE 15.6. Causes of delirium and confusion in the elderly

Central nervous system (CNS) causes
CNS degenerative diseases
Seizure and postictal states
Stroke
Primary or metastatic tumor
Subdural hematoma or CNS injury
Meningitis or encephalitis
Arteritis

Metabolic/peripheral causes
Hypothermia
Hypoxia and decreased perfusion (congestive heart failure, anemia, pulmonary embolism)
Medication side effects (sedating drugs, antihistamines, beta blockers, opiates, etc.)

Sepsis and infections
Pneumonia
Urinary tract infections
Gastrointestinal infections
Wound infections

Other causes
Alcohol
Renal failure
Malignancy
Liver failure
Electrolyte disturbances
Anesthesia
Endocrine-hypoglycemia, hyperglycemia, hypothyroidism, hyperthyroidism
Sleep deprivation
Acute psychosis

Adapted from ref. [12].

A careful history may establish a temporal relationship between specific events and symptoms. This is generally the most helpful item in the practitioner's armamentarium to assist in arriving at a diagnosis. A careful review of medications is vital. The clinician must consider medication side effect as a possible cause of any new symptom in the geriatric patient. Over-the-counter medications, supplements, herbal preparations, as well as home remedies should be discussed. Many geriatric patients do not consider these nonprescribed treatments as bona-fide "medication." Abrupt discontinuation of some medications can create confusion and anxiety-like behaviors in the elderly [16]. This is common with benzodiazepine therapy but could also occur with other medications. Alcohol withdrawal may produce symptoms of irritability and tremulousness in mild cases and delirium tremens in severe cases [17]. Changes in drug metabolism may result in delirium, warranting close attention by the practitioner to medication doses [18] and drug–drug interactions.

In the evaluation of delirium, the practitioner should perform a careful history and a thorough physical examination. Particular attention should be paid to the neurological exam. Laboratory tests, head computed tomography (CT), lumbar puncture, and electroencephalogram (EEG) are useful in many cases.

In summary, delirium may be a common event in elderly patients. Some symptoms of delirium may present as an anxiety disorder. On the other hand, elderly patients with an anxiety disorder may present with symptoms of a delirium state. The primary care practitioner will be better able to discern the correct diagnosis by taking an accurate, complete history and performing a physical examination, followed by appropriate testing as indicated.

TREATMENT

Medication Compliance

In prescribing any medication for the geriatric patient, the practitioner must evaluate the patient's cognition and ability to take medications as prescribed. If the geriatric patient requires medication to control anxiety, depression, or any psychiatric disorder, the practitioner should assess the issues listed in Table 15.7.

The Institute of Medicine reports medication nonadherence as a notable source of medical errors [19]. Medications are only effective when the dosage regimen is followed as prescribed. The geriatric patient is at risk for overdosing or underdosing. Taking the time to evaluate the geriatric patient's compliance with medication will facilitate improved treatment outcome.

TABLE 15.7. Medication compliance issues in the elderly

Does the patient bring medication to the office visit?
Does the patient use a pill organizer?
Is there someone else living in the home to assist with dosage?
Is there a caregiver (e.g., home health aid or personal caregiver) who
    visits on a routine basis?
Is there a need to request home health/personal care evaluation?
Is there affordable electronic monitoring to assist with dosage compliance?

Medical Therapy

Benzodiazepines

About half of elderly patients with a diagnosis of anxiety disorder
are treated by a pharmacological intervention [11]. The benzodiazepines are the most frequently prescribed class of drug therapy
[11]. Despite the common use of benzodiazepines in the treatment
of geriatric anxiety, few randomized controlled trials exist to sub-
stantiate their use. The common consensus is that benzodiazepines
are effective medications in the elderly, but should be used with a
degree of caution. The benzodiazepines have a sedative effect that
may worsen cognition in the elderly. The use of lower doses and a
frequent reassessment of elderly patients being treated with benzodiazepines are recommended.

There are numerous benzodiazepines available on the market
for the treatment of anxiety symptoms. A general recommendation
is that shorter half-life benzodiazepines be used when treating the
elderly. Longer acting benzodiazepines may not clear from the
system as quickly in geriatric patients and, hence, tend to accumulate, causing oversedation. Table 15.8 lists several benzodiazepines
that are useful in treating anxiety symptoms [21].

Selective Serotonin Reuptake Inhibitors

Despite reports that the selective serotonin reuptake inhibitors
(SSRIs) may cause a slight increased initial risk of suicide in the
elderly [20], there is considerable recognition that this class of
medication is quite helpful in the management of anxiety disorders. The effect of SSRI treatment is not as immediate as that seen
with benzodiazepine therapy. An SSRI may require 7 to 30 days
to reach a desired effect [21]. Starting with a low dose is recommended in the elderly, perhaps half of the usual staring dose for
a younger adult patient [21]. In general, these medications have a
relatively long half-life and may take as long as 30 days to reach
steady state [21].

TABLE 15.8. Benzodiazepines

Drug name	Available dosages	Half-life	Active metabolite (half-life)	Daily maximum dose	Starting dose
Alprazolam (Xanax)	0.25 mg 0.5 mg 1 mg 2 mg	6–27 hours, average 11–12 hours	No active metabolite	4 mg/day for GAD 6 mg/day for PD (Rec.: 2 mg maximum in elderly) dose	0.25 mg t.i.d. (q.d. or b.i.d. in elderly)
Alprazolam (Xanax XR)	0.5 mg 1 mg 2 mg 3 mg	Average 11–12 hours	No active metabolite	6 mg/day (Rec.: 2 mg/day in elderly)	0.5 mg q.d.
Clonazepam (Klonopin)	0.5 mg 1 mg 2 mg	18–50 hours, average 30–40 hours	No active metabolite	4 mg/day (Rec.: 2 mg maximum dose in elderly)	0.25 mg b.i.d. (q.d. in elderly)
Chlordiaze-poxide (Librium)	5 mg 10 mg 25 mg	24–48 hours	Desmethyldiazepam (30–200 hours) Oxazepam (3–21 hours) Demoxepam (14–95 hours) Desmethylchlor-diazepoxide (18 hours)	100 mg/day (Rec.: 20 mg maximum dose in elderly)	5 mg b.i.d.
Clorazepate (Tranxene)	3.75 mg 7.5 mg 15 mg SD 22.5 mg SD-half 11.25 mg	Pro-drug average 48 hours	Oxazepam (3–21 hours) Desmethyldiazepam (30–200 hours)	60 mg/day (Rec.: 15 mg maximum dose in elderly)	7.5 mg q.d. (3.75 mg q.d. in elderly) 11.25 q.d.

Continued

TABLE 15.8. (continued)

Drug name	Available dosages	Half-life	Active metabolite (half-life)	Daily maximum dose	Starting dose
Diazepam (Valium)	2 mg 5 mg 10 mg	20–80 hours	Desmethyldiazepam (30–200 hours) Oxazepam (3–21 hours) 3-Hydroxydiazepam (5–20 hours)	40 mg/day (Rec.: <10 mg maximum dose in elderly)	2 mg t.i.d. (2 mg q.d. in elderly)
Oxazepam (Serax)	10 mg 15 mg 30 mg	3–21 hours	No active metabolite	30 mg/day (Rec.: 15 mg/day in elderly)	10 mg q.d.
Lorazepam (Ativan)	0.5 mg 1 mg 2 mg	12 hours	No active metabolite	6 mg/day (Rec.: 2 mg/day in elderly)	0.5 mg t.i.d. (0.5 mg q.d. in elderly)

GAD, generalized anxiety disorder; PD, panic disorder; Rec., recommended; SD, single dose. Adapted from ref. [21].

Long-term use of SSRIs in the elderly has been shown to be effective and safe [3]. Side effects are usually mild at lower doses. The elderly patient may be more sensitive to medications in general, and the SSRIs are no exception. Side effects of SSRI use in the geriatric patient are listed in Table 15.9 [22].

A discontinuation syndrome is possible following long-term treatment with this class of medicine. The syndrome is manifested by several symptoms including increased agitation, multiple somatic sensations such as tingling and electrical shocks, and a general feeling of illness. The SSRIs with shorter half-lives are more likely to cause this problem. Tapering of the dose over 1 to 2 weeks will reduce or prevent the discontinuation syndrome (Table 15.10).

TABLE 15.9. SSRI side effects in the geriatric patient

• Dry mouth	• Constipation
• Decreased libido/delayed ejaculation	• Overstimulation
• Weight gain	• Initial suicide risk

Adapted from refs. [20] and [22].

TABLE 15.10. SSRI serotonin reuptake inhibitors

Drug name	Available dosages	Half-life	Daily maximum dose	Starting dose
Fluoxetine (Prozac)	10 mg 20 mg 90 mg (weekly)	48–72 hours	60 mg/day (Rec.: 20 mg/day in elderly)	10 mg q.d.
Sertraline (Zoloft)	25 mg 50 mg 100 mg	26 hours	200 mg/day (Rec.: 100 mg/ day in elderly)	25 mg q.d.
Paroxetine (Paxil) (Paxil CR)	Paxil 10 mg 20 mg 30 mg 40 mg CR 12.5 mg 25 mg 37.5 mg	21 hours	60 mg/day (Rec.: 30 mg/day in elderly) 75 mg/day (Rec.: 25 mg/ day in elderly)	10 mg q.d. 12.5 mg q.d.
Citalopram (Celexa)	10 mg 20 mg 40 mg (liquid)	35 hours	60 mg/day (Rec.: 30 mg/day in elderly)	10 mg q.d.
Escitalopram (Lexapro)	5 mg 10 mg 20 mg (liquid)		20 mg/day (Rec.: 10 mg/day in elderly)	5 mg q.d.
Fluvoxamine (Luvox)	25 mg 50 mg 100 mg	15.6 hours	300 mg/day (Rec.: 150 mg/ day in elderly)	25 mg q.d.

Adapted from ref. [21].

Tricyclic Antidepressants

Tricyclic antidepressant medications (TCAs) have been available for many years. Prior to the introduction of the SSRIs in the 1980s, this class of medication was the backbone of anxiety and depression therapy. The TCAs are still a useful treatment for the elderly patient, but side effects preclude their common use given newer, better tolerated medications. As with almost all other medications in the elderly, it is wise to "start low and go slow" when dosing TCAs. The same rule of thumb applies as for the SSRIs (i.e., start with about half of the dose normally prescribed for a younger patient). Close follow-up and monitoring of the patient for side effects, especially at the initiation of therapy, is strongly advised. Side effects include those listed in Table 15.11 [22].

Table 15.12 lists some TCAs used in the elderly patient with anxiety and depression.

Other Medication Treatment Options

There are other classes of medication used in the treatment of geriatric anxiety disorders. Buspirone (BuSpar), an azapirone, may be helpful in the treatment of anxiety in the elderly [21]. Buspirone is not an SSRI, TCA, or benzodiazepine. It is indicated for the symptoms of generalized anxiety disorder. Side effects include headache, dizziness, light-headedness, excitation, and nausea. The usual staring dose is 5 mg t.i.d. It may be increased to a maximum of 60 mg/day, usually prescribed as 20 mg t.i.d.

Hydroxyzine (Vistaril, Atarax) is an antihistamine compound with sedative-like qualities. It is not considered first-line therapy for anxiety [21]. Hydroxyzine may produce considerable sedation, dry mouth, and constipation. It is relatively inexpensive, but its side effects preclude its widespread use in the elderly. Hydroxyzine pamoate (Vistaril) is usually started at 25 mg at h.s. and may be increased to as much as 100 mg q.d.

The serotonin-norepinephrine reuptake inhibitors (SNRIs) are a unique class of medication that affect both serotonin and

TABLE 15.11. Side effect of tricyclic antidepressants in the geriatric patient

• Dry mouth	• Constipation
• Urinary retention	• Sedation
• Orthostatic hypotension	• Weight gain

Adapted from ref. [22].

TABLE 15.12. Tricyclic antidepressants

Drug name	Available dosages	Daily maximum dose	Starting dose	FDA-approved indication	Serotonin affinity	Norepine-phrine affinity	Dopamine affinity
Amitriptyline (Elavil)	10 mg 25 mg 50 mg 75 mg 100 mg 150 mg	300 mg/day (Rec.: 100 mg/day in elderly)	10–25 mg q.h.s.	Depression	4+	4+	0
Nortriptyline (Pamelor)	10 mg 25 mg 50 mg 75 mg	150 mg/day (Rec.: 50 mg/day in elderly)	10 mg q.h.s.	Depression	2+	3+	0
Doxepin (Sinequan)	10 mg 25 mg 50 mg 75 mg 100 mg 150 mg	300 mg/day (Rec.: <100 mg/day in elderly)	25 mg q.h.s.	Depression, anxiety	3+	1+	0
Clomipramine (Anafranil)	25 mg 50 mg 75 mg	250 mg/day (Rec.: <100 mg/day in lderly)	25 mg q.h.s.	Obsessive-compulsive disorder	3+	2+	0
Imipramine (Tofranil)	10 mg 25 mg 50 mg	300 mg/day (Rec.: <100 mg/day in elderly)	10 mg q.h.s.	Depression	3+	2+	0

Adapted from ref. [21].

norepinephrine reuptake. These medications include duloxetine (Cymbalta) and venlafaxine (Effexor, Effexor XR). Both Effexor XR and Cymbalta are approved by the U.S. Food and Drug Administration for use in generalized anxiety disorder. Both are effective in treating depression as well. These medications have usefulness in the treatment of anxiety symptoms in the elderly [23–25]. Table 15.13 lists available SNRI medications and therapeutic dosages.

Cognitive Behavior Therapy

Cognitive behavior therapy involves cognitive restructuring of responses, inherent or learned, that lead to an anxiety response. For instance, a patient with panic disorder may have developed a response to a perceived threat to safety and security that is counterproductive to their well-being. The response may trigger a panic attack or severe anxiety symptoms. An elderly patient may present with symptoms of a panic attack as listed in Table 15.14.

These symptoms are distressful and frightening to patients. Geriatric patients, because of age, frailty, illness, or disability, may not be able to distinguish the panic attack symptoms from those of a cardiac or neurological disease. The role of cognitive behavior therapy is to work with the patient to restructure thoughts and relearn behaviors that allow the patient to gain a sense of comfort and security. The ultimate goal is to have the patient gain a sense of control.

The primary care practitioner may provide cognitive behavioral therapy. Time demands of a primary care practice may not allow much opportunity for such an intervention. In some instances, the primary care practitioner may prefer to manage the treatment with medications and refer the patient to a therapist experienced in cognitive behavioral therapy.

Combined cognitive behavioral therapy and medical therapy has been shown to improve treatment outcome [25]. This dual-faceted approach has become an accepted and reliable way to treat anxiety symptoms.

TABLE 15.13. Selective serotonin-norepinephrine reuptake inhibitors

Drug name	Available dosages	Daily maximum dose	Starting dose	FDA-approved indication	Half-life	Serotonin receptor affinity (0-4)	Norepinephrine receptor affinity (0-4)
Duloxetine (Cymbalta)	20 mg 30 mg 60 mg	60 mg	20 mg or 30 mg	Major depression generalized anxiety disorder, neuropathic pain	12 hours	4+	4+
Venlafaxine (Effexor)	25 mg 37.5 mg 50 mg 75 mg 100 mg	225 mg	25 mg	Major depression	5 hours for venlafaxine; 11 hours for active metabolite	4+	3+
Venlafaxine (Effexor XR)	37.5 mg 75 mg 150 mg	225 mg	37.5 mg	Major depression, general anxiety disorder, social anxiety disorder	5 hours for venlafaxine; 11 hours for active metabolite	4+	3+

Adapted from ref. [21].

TABLE 15.14. Symptoms of a panic attack in the geriatric patient

- Palpitations, pounding heart, increased heart rate
- Overwhelming feeling of doom, fear of dying
- Sweating
- Sensation of shortness of breath or smothering
- Sensation of choking or blocked airway
- Feeling dizzy, lightheaded, faint or fading away
- Chills or hot flashes
- Fear of losing control or "going crazy"
- Chest pain, discomfort, pressure
- Feelings of unreality
- Numbness or tingling of hands, feet, or lips

Adapted from ref. [25].

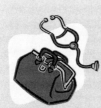

Pearls for the Practitioner

- Always remember to ask the elderly patient about any treatment that is being administered by another practitioner. Many practitioners in primary care know their patients quite well. Despite this fact, some patients may see other practitioners, consult a specialist, or see another practitioner while traveling. Despite the best of intentions, a patient may not volunteer that a new medication has been prescribed by another practitioner or that a medically significant event (i.e., injury, minor surgery, or outpatient procedure) has occurred and has a major impact on health care management.
- Over-the-counter medications and herbal supplements pose a serious problem for the health care management of elderly patients. Aspirin may interfere with anticoagulation drug treatment. Antihistamines may cause constipation, urinary retention, sedation, and decreased secretions in elderly patients. Ibuprofen and naproxen produce a degree of sodium and water retention as well as gastric inflammation and diarrhea. All of these over-the-counter medications and others may be used on a frequent basis by elderly patients. The practitioner should periodically review the use of over-the-counter medicines with each patient.

- Always address the elderly patient in clear speech tones. Loss of hearing is common in the elderly. This fact does not necessarily warrant the practitioner's loud voice. Many older patients express a concern that the practitioner is angry because they were subjected to loud explanations and questioning during the clinic visit. Patients complain that the practitioner made them feel stupid by such behavior and become offended. The practitioner should not always assume that advanced age is associated with presbyacusis (loss of ability to perceive or discriminate sounds as a part of the aging process) or a lack of medical sophistication.

- Many elderly patients may not adhere to all the recommendations of the practitioner. This is not necessarily a sign of disrespect. As with any patient in any adult age group, acceptance of treatment may be difficult for some. There may be a misconception about why a particular medication is being prescribed and what outcome is expected. Some elderly patients believe that "if one is good, two is better." Unintentional overdose may result. It is inherent upon the practitioner to give the elderly patient a clear, concise description of the medication. Asking the patient to repeat back to the practitioner what has just been instructed can provide the practitioner a gauge of the elderly patient's understanding of treatment. A simple nod of the head may be a false representation of the patient's understanding of the diagnosis and therapy.

- Many elderly patients are on a fixed income. The cost of prescription medications continues to rise. Simply purchasing the prescription medicine may be out of reach for some patients. In some cases, the patient may purchase the medicine only to take less than the prescribed dose in order to "stretch out the prescription." Sample medications are helpful and appreciated by most elderly patients. Providing samples also gives the elderly patient a sense of value to the health care visit.

- Listen and learn from the elderly patient. The elderly have lived a lifetime of experiences that often supersede those life experiences of the practitioner. It is wise for the practitioner to be respectful of such experience. Often, simply acknowledging the elderly patient's many years of "hard knocks" allows the practitioner to gain a greater rapport. Once established, this rapport allows the practitioner to have

Continued

Continued

a keener sense of awareness of untoward disease symptoms, drug side effects, and important medical history details that might not otherwise be recognized or voiced.

- Visual impairment is a common ailment of the elderly. Reading prescription label instructions, measuring doses, taking the correct medicine at the correct time are all vision dependent functions. A little white pill for one condition may be easily confused with another little white pill for another entirely different condition. Reminding the patient to double-check medication prior to consumption may help avoid errors in treatment. Usually the pharmacist can offer aids for visually impaired patients that reduce the chance of medication error.

- The practitioner may fully and easily understand the reason for medical treatment, but many elderly patients may not. Keeping dosing schedules simple and less complicated may improve compliance. If memory impairment is an issue for a particular patient, asking a family member or caregiver to help administer medication is a helpful strategy. A simple explanation using common language terms may help the elderly patient understand the treatment as well as the practitioner's rationale for using a particular drug therapy. Many elderly patients are capable of understanding instructions and are interested in the treatment being prescribed for them if explained in understandable terms.

- Many elderly patients experience gastrointestinal dysfunction that may involve decreased esophageal motility. This condition may be made worse by stroke, achalasia, esophageal stricture, and decreased salivation. Large pills and capsules may be difficult or impossible to swallow. The practitioner should keep this in mind when prescribing any medication for elderly patients with swallowing impairment.

- As with many other treatment modalities in the elderly, psychotropic medications should be started at a low dose. The "start low and go slow" concept is always wise, especially in the elderly. The expected effect from a prescribed psychotropic medication may not be immediately apparent. Some medications require days or several weeks to reach full effect. A relatively low dose of a medication may actually be the correct dose for an elderly patient; therefore, it is wise for the practitioner to be patient and allow time for the treatment to take effect.

- Many elderly patients require the assistance of a caregiver. Often the caregiver is a family member, or a friend, neighbor, or hired individual. While the issue of health care information confidentiality cannot be minimized, at times the practitioner must address diagnosis and treatment of an elderly patient with another person present such as a caregiver or family member. There may be occasions when the caregiver or family member is a tremendous help in areas such as clarifying history and understanding treatment instructions. Despite this fact, it is imperative for the practitioner to speak directly with the elderly patient and remember that the patient, not the caregiver or family member, is the practitioner's primary focus.

References

1. U.S. Department of Health and Human Services, Administration on Aging. A Profile of Older Americans. Washington, DC: DHHS, 2005.
2. Lundberg M, Larsson M, Ostlund H, Styf J. Kinesiophobia among patients with musculoskeletal pain in primary healthcare. J Rehabil Med 2006;38:37–43.
3. Reynolds C, et al. Maintenance treatment of major depression in old age. N Engl J Med 2006;354:1130–1138.
4. Smalbrugge M, Pot AM, Jongenelis L, Gundy CM, Beekman AT, Eefsting JA. The impact of depression and anxiety on well being, disability and use of health care services in nursing home patients. Int J Geriatr Psychiatry 2006;21(4):325–332.
5. Janicak P, Davis J, Preskorn S, Ayd F. Principles and Practice of Psychopharmacotherapy. Baltimore, MD: Williams & Wilkins, 1993: 481–536.
6. Benet L, Mitchell J, Sheiner L. Pharmacokinetics: the dynamics of drug absorption, distribution, and elimination. In: Goodman A, Gilman A, Rall T, Nies A, Taylor P, eds. The Pharmacologic Basis of Therapeutics. Elmsford, NY: Pergamon Press, 1990:3–48.
7. Jones J. Drugs and the elderly. In: Clinical Aspects of Aging. Baltimore, MD: Williams & Wilkins, 1989:41–60.
8. Streiner D, Cairney J, Veldhuizen S. The epidemiology of psychological problems in the elderly. Can J Psychiatry 2006; 51(3):185–191.
9. Beekman A, et al. Anxiety Disorders in later life: a report from the Longitudinal Aging Study, Amsterdam. Int J Geriatr Psychiatry 1998;13(10):717–726.
10. Himmelfarb S, Murrell S. The prevalence and correlates of anxiety symptoms on older adults. J Psychol 1984;116:159–167.

11. Ayers C, Wetherell J, Stanley M. Treating late-life anxiety. Psych Times 2006;March:17–26.

12. Blazer D. Depression. In: Abrams W, Berkow R, eds. The Merck Manual Of Geriatrics. Rahway, NJ: Merck, 1990:1014–1018.

13. Rayner A, O'Brien J, Shoenbachler B. Behavior disorders of dementia: recognition and treatment. Am Fam Physician 2006;73(4):647–652.

14. Wells C. Pseudodementia. Am J Psychiatry 1979;136:895.

15. Folstein M, et al. Mini-mental state: a practical method for grading the cognitive state of patients for the clinician. J Psychiatr Res 1975;12:189.

16. Yamada K, Awadalla S. Neurologic disorders. In: Green G, Harris I, Lin G, Moylan K, eds. The Washington Manual of Medical Therapeutics. Philadelphia: Lippincott Williams & Wilkins, 2004:531–537.

17. Gaudreau J, Gagnon P, et al. Psychoactive medications and risk of delirium in hospitalized cancer patients. J Clin Oncol 2005;23(27):6712–6718.

18. White S, Calver B, Newsday V, et al. Enzymes of drug metabolism during delirium. Age Ageing 2005;34(6):603–608.

19. Ownby R, Hertzog C, Crocco E, Duara R. Factors related to medication adherence in memory disorder clinic patients. Aging Ment Health 2006;10(4):378–385.

20. Juurlink D, et al. The risk of suicide with selective serotonin reuptake inhibitors in the elderly. Am J Psychiatry 2006;163:813–821.

21. DeBattista C, Schatzberg A. 2003 Psychotropic dosing and monitoring guidelines. Primary Psychiatry 2003;10(7):80–84, 87–96.

22. Culpepper L. Identifying and treating panic disorder in primary care. J Clin Psychiatry 2004;65(suppl 5):1–23.

23. Gliatto M. Generalized anxiety disorder. Am Fam Physician 2000;62(7):1048–1061.

24. Gale C, Oakley-Bowne M. Generalized anxiety disorder. In: Tovey D, ed. Clinical Evidence, vol. 14. London: BMJ Publishing Group, 2005:334–336.

25. Otto M, Deveney C. Cognitive behavioral therapy and the treatment of panic disorder: efficacy and strategies. J Clin Psychiatry 2005;66(suppl 4):28–32.

Anxiety Disorders Resources

(Note: the TDD/TTY telephone numbers are for telecommunication devices for the deaf.)

Agoraphobics Building Independent Lives
400 West 32nd Street
Richmond, VA 23225
(804) 353-3964
www.anxietysupport.org

American Association of Suicidology
5221 Wisconsin Avenue, NW
Washington, DC 20015
202-237-2280
National Suicide Prevention Lifeline 1-800-273-TALK (8255)
www.suicidology.org

American Foundation for Suicide Prevention
120 Wall Street, 22nd floor
New York, NY 10005
212-363-3500
888-333-AFSP (2377) Toll-Free
www.afsp.org

American Psychiatric Association
1000 Wilson Boulevard, Suite 1825
Arlington, VA 22209-3901
703-907-7300
www.psych.org

American Psychological Association
750 First Street, N.E.
Washington, DC 20002-4242
800-374-2721
202-336-5500
TDD/TTY: 202-336-6213
www.apa.org

Anxiety Disorders Association of America
8730 Georgia Avenue, Suite 600
Silver Spring, MD 20910
240-485-1001
www.adaa.org

Association for Behavioral and Cognitive Therapies
305 Seventh Avenue, 16th floor
New York, NY 10001
(212) 647-1890
www.aabt.org

Doctors Guide
www.docguide.com

Freedom from Fear
308 Seaview Avenue
Staten Island, NY 10305
718-351-1717
www.freedomfromfear.org

International Society for Traumatic Stress Studies
60 Revere Drive, Suite 500
Northbrook IL 60062
847-480-9028
www.istss.org

MedlinePlus: Health Information
www.medlineplus.gov

Mental Health America (formerly National Mental Health Association)
2000 N. Beauregard St., 6t floor
Alexandria, VA 22311
800-969-6MHA (6642)
703-684-7722
TTY: 800-433-5959
www.mentalhealthamerica.net

National Alliance for the Mentally Ill
Colonial Place Three
2107 Wilson Boulevard, Suite 300
Arlington, VA 22201-3042
800-950-NAMI (6264)
703-524-7600
TDD: 703-516-7227
www.nami.org

National Anxiety Foundation
3135 Custer Drive
Lexington, KY 40517-4001
606-272-7166

National Center for Posttraumatic Stress Disorder
U.S. Department of Veterans Affairs
VA Medical Center (116D)
215 N. Main Street
White River Junction, VT 05009
(802) 296-6300
www.ncptsd.org

National Clearinghouse for Alcohol and Drug Information
P.O. Box 2345
Rockville, MD 20847-2345
800-729-6686
301-468-2600
www.health.org

National Drug Abuse Information and Treatment Referral
Hot Line and National Institute on Drug Abuse Help Line
12280 Wilkins Avenue
Rockville, MD 20852
800-662-HELP (4357)
800-66-AYUDA (Spanish-speaking callers)

National Institute of Mental Health
Public Information Communications Branch
6001 Executive Boulevard, Room 8184, MSC 9663
Bethesda, MD 20892-9663
1-866-615-6464 Toll-Free
301-443-4513
TTY: 1-866-415-8051 Toll-Free
TTY: 301-443-8431
www.nimh.nih.gov

National Mental Health Consumers' Self-Help Clearinghouse
1211 Chestnut Street, Suite 1207
Philadelphia, PA 19107
800-553-4539
215 751-1810
www.mhselfhelp.org

National Mental Health Information Center
Substance Abuse and Mental Health Services Administration
P.O. Box 42557
Washington, DC 20015
800-789-2647
TDD: 866-889-2647
www.mentalhealth.org

Obsessive-Compulsive Foundation, Inc.
676 State Street
New Haven, CT 06511
203-401-2070
www.ocfoundation.org

Phobics Anonymous
World Service Headquarters
P.O.Box 1180
Palm Springs, CA 92263
760-332-COPE (2673)
www.healsocialanxiety.com

PTSD Alliance
www.ptsdalliance.org

Sidran Institute
www.sidran.org

Substance Abuse and Mental Health Services Administration
1 Choke Cherry Road
Room 8-1036
Rockville, MD
800-662-HELP (4357)
www.samhsa.gov

TERRAP (TERRitorial APprehension)
648 Menlo Avenue, Suite 5
Menlo Park, CA 94025
415-327-1312
www.terrap.com

Glossary

This glossary is designed to assist primary care practitioners and other non psychiatrists with mental health terminology, particularly relating to the anxiety disorders. Psychiatry is an evolving, complex science and the area of anxiety disorders is no exception. To assist the practitioner to better understand and thus become more comfortable with the anxiety disorders, as well as to keep updated, we adapted a practical glossary from several excellent mental health resources to facilitate everyday primary care practice (1–7). This pocket guide glossary is a concise, easy to understand resource for the practitioner requiring a quick reference for writing a patient history and mental status examination, formulating a diagnosis, educating patients and their families about anxiety disorders, and discussing patients in consultation. We encourage the reader to refer to pertinent Internet sites and other resources for a more comprehensive listing of mental health terminology.

acetylcholine Neurotransmitter that helps to regulate memory and control actions of skeletal and smooth muscle.

achluophobia Fear of darkness.

acrophobia Fear of heights.

acute posttraumatic stress disorder Posttraumatic stress disorder that lasts from 1 to 3 months.

acute stress disorder Anxiety disorder that develops following exposure to a traumatic event, lasts 1 month or less, and is characterized by reexperiencing the trauma, and experiencing dissociative symptoms, increased arousal, and avoidance.

adrenergic system System of organs and nerves in which catecholamines such as dopamine, epinephrine, and norepinephrine are the neurotransmitters.

aerophagia Excessive swallowing of air.

aerophobia Fear of flying.

affect Behavior that expresses a subjectively experienced emotion. Manifestations may include constricted, labile, blunted, flat, appropriate, or inappropriate.

agitation Severe anxiety associated with motor restlessness. Examples include fidgeting, pacing, and wringing of hands.

agonist Drug that mimics the action of a natural chemical messenger within the body by occupying cell receptors.

agoraphobia Fear of open spaces or leaving the familiar setting of home.

alexithymia Inability or difficulty in describing or being aware of one's emotions or moods and a limited fantasy life.

algophobia Fear of pain.

amathophobia Fear of dust.

amaxophobia Fear of riding in a car

antianxiety medications See *anxiolytics*.

anticholinergic effects Interference with the action of acetylcholine in the brain and the peripheral nervous system by any drug that may result in symptoms such as dry mouth, blurred vision, constipation, and decreased ability to urinate.

antidepressants Medications used in the treatment of depression, generalized anxiety disorder, panic disorder, obsessive-compulsive disorder, social anxiety disorder, posttraumatic stress disorder, premenstrual dysphoric disorder, attention-deficit/hyperactivity disorder, chronic pain, and other disorders. The mechanism of action of antidepressant medications appears to be due to effects on pre- and postsynaptic receptors affecting the release and reuptake of brain neurotransmitters.

antihistamines Medications used to minimize or prevent the action of histamine. Antihistamines are useful as sedatives, hypnotics, and may be used to reduce anxiety symptoms in patients with mild symptoms.

anxiety Feeling of apprehension, tension, or uneasiness often marked by physical symptoms, caused by anticipation of danger, the source of which is largely unknown or unrecognized. May be regarded as pathological when it interferes with social and occupational functioning, achievement of desired goals, or emotional comfort.

anxiety hysteria Early psychoanalytic term for what is now called phobia.

anxiety neurosis See *neurosis*.

anxiolytics Medications used to relieve emotional tension.

astrapophobia Fear of lightening.

autophobia Fear of being alone.

autonomic nervous system Part of the peripheral nervous system that regulates the involuntary body actions such as breathing, blood pressure, heart rate, and pupil dilation; also regulates the flight or fight response.

aviophobia Fear of flying.

axon Fiberlike extension of a neuron through which information exits to the target cells.

bathophobia Fear of depths.

behavior Sum total of the psyche that includes impulses, wishes, drives, motivation, instincts, and cravings that are expressed by a persons behavior or motor activity.

behavior therapy Treatment used to help patients substitute desirable or healthier responses and behavior patterns for undesirable or maladaptive ones. The basic techniques include behavior modification, operant conditioning, systematic desensitization, shaping, token economy, relaxation training, aversion training, exposure therapy, flooding, modeling, paradoxical intention, and social skills training.

benzodiazepines Class of medications that have potent hypnotic, sedative, and anxiolytic effects; also called antianxiety medications or anxiolytics.

beta-blockers Class of medications that inhibits the action of β-adrenergic receptors, which modulate cardiac and respiratory functions, and the dilation and constriction of blood vessels. Prescribed to ease physical symptoms of anxiety.

biogenic amines Organic substances subdivided into catecholamines (epinephrine, norepinephrine, dopamine) and indoleamines (tryptophan, serotonin).

chronic posttraumatic stress disorder Posttraumatic stress disorder that lasts longer than 3 months.

claustrophobia Fear of enclosed or confining spaces.

cognition Awareness with perception, intuition, judgment, and memory as well as the mental process by which knowledge is acquired.

cognitive-behavioral therapy Form of psychotherapy focused on changing thoughts and behaviors that are related to specific target symptoms and aimed at symptom reduction and improved functioning.

cognitive therapy Treatment approach based on the theory that our cognitions or thoughts control a large part of our behaviors and emotions. Changing the way we think can result in positive changes in the way we act and feel.

comorbidity Simultaneous appearance of two or more illnesses in the same individual.

compulsion Repetitive ritualistic behavior or thoughts to prevent or reduce distress or to prevent a dreaded event or situation.

conditioning Psychological modification of responses to stimuli to establish new behavior.

corticotropin-releasing factor (CRF) Substance synthesized in the hypothalamus that regulates the secretion of adrenocorticotropic hormone (ACTH) from the posterior pituitary. Effects include activation of the sympathetic nervous system and regulation of behavioral responses to stress.

cortisol A steroid hormone produced in the adrenal glands responsible for many of the physiological effects of stress.

cynophobia Fear of dogs.

cytochrome P-450 Enzyme system in the liver and small intestine that plays a key role in medication metabolism.

dendrite Branch of a nerve cell that receives nerve impulses from the axon of a neighboring nerve.

derealization Feeling of estrangement or detachment from ones environment.

Diagnostic and Statistical Manual of Mental Disorders (**DSM**) The American Psychiatric Association's official classification of mental disorders.

didaskaleinophobia Fear of going to school.

differential diagnosis Process whereby multiple possible disorders are considered to formulate a final diagnosis.

distractibility Inability to maintain attention.

dopamine Neurotransmitter associated with movement, attention, motivation, learning, and the brain's pleasure and reward system.

dread Pervasive anxiety usually related to a specific danger.

emotion Complex feeling state often accompanied by physiological changes. External manifestation of emotion is affect.

epinephrine Catecholamine, also known as adrenalin, secreted by the adrenal gland and by neurons of the sympathetic nervous system. Responsible for many of the physical manifestations of fear and anxiety.

eremophobia Fear of being alone.

erythrophobia Fear of blushing.

exposure therapy Method of therapy that involves gradually exposing patients to a feared object or situation. Patients learn that the object or situation can be faced and that avoidance is unnecessary.

fatigue Feeling of sleepiness, weariness, or irritability after a period of mental or bodily activity.

fear Unpleasant emotional and physiological state in response to a realistic threat or danger.

flooding (implosion) A behavior therapy procedure in which the causes of the anxiety are intensely presented either in real life or in imagination. The desensitizers are continued until the stimuli no longer produce disabling anxiety.

free-floating anxiety Generalized anxiety that is severe and persistent and not attached to any particular object, idea, or event.

frigophobia Fear of cold weather.

γ-aminobutyric acid (GABA) Major inhibitory neurotransmitter in the brain.

generalized anxiety disorder Excessive and unrealistic worry about many life circumstances, unrelated to another illness.

gephyrophobia Fear of crossing bridges.

global assessment of functioning Numerical assessment of the patient's overall symptomatology and psychological, social, and occupational functioning. A hypothetical continuum of mental health-illness, on a scale of 1 to 100, with 100 being the highest score.

globus hystericus Disturbing sensation of a lump in the throat.

glutamate Excitatory amino acid in the brain.

gynophobia Fear of women.

5-HIAA (5 hydroxyindoleacetic acid) Major metabolite of serotonin.

hippocampus Brain structure involved in learning, memory, and emotion.

homophobia Fear of homosexual persons.

homovanillic acid (HVA) Principal metabolite of dopamine.

hydrophobia Fear of water.

hyperventilation Overbreathing marked by reduction of blood carbon dioxide.

hypothalamus Complex brain structure composed of many nuclei with various functions. The head ganglion of the autonomic nervous system. Functions include control of heart rate, blood pressure, respiration, and fight or flight response.

incidence Number of new cases of a disorder that occur during a specific time period.

indoleamine One of a group of biogenic amines such as serotonin.

inducer Drug or substance that increases an enzyme's ability to metabolize a substrate.

inhibitor Drug or substance that prevents an enzyme from metabolizing a substrate.

initial insomnia Difficulty falling asleep.

insomnia A dyssomnia consisting of difficulty initiating or maintaining sleep or of nonrestorative sleep associated with daytime fatigue or impaired daytime functioning.

International Classification of Diseases (ICD) Official list of disease categories issued by the World Health Organization.

kakorrhaphiophobia Fear of failure.

katagelophobia Fear of ridicule.

keraunophobia Fear of thunder.

locus ceruleus Small area in the brainstem containing norepinephrine neurons.

logophobia Fear of words.

MHPG (3-methoxy-4-hydroxyphenylglycol) Major metabolite of brain norepinephrine excreted in the urine.

middle insomnia Waking up after falling asleep without difficulty and then having difficulty in falling asleep again.

mood Pervasive and sustained feeling tone that is experienced internally.

musophobia Fear of mice.

mysophobia Fear of dirt and germs.

needle phobia Intense, persistent, pathological fear of receiving an injection.

nervous breakdown Nonspecific, nonmedical term for a mental disorder.

neurasthenia Disorder in ICD-10, characterized by persisting complaints of physical and mental weakness or fatigue after performing daily activities and inability to recover with normal periods of rest. Typical symptoms include dizziness, tension headaches, muscular aches and pains, irritability, and sleep problems.

neurochemistry Branch of chemistry dealing with the nervous system, including chemical components, passage of impulses through the nerve cell, and transmission across synapses.

neuroendocrinology Science regarding the relationship between the nervous system and the endocrine system, particularly the hypothalamus, which stimulates or inhibits the pituitary's secretion of hormones.

neurohormone Chemical messenger usually produced within the hypothalamus, carried to the pituitary and then to other central nervous system cells. Neurohormones interact with a variety of cells, whereas neurotransmitters interact with other neurons.

neuroimaging General term referring to technologies such as computed tomography (CT), single photon emission computed tomography (SPECT), magnetic resonance tomography (MRI), and positron emission tomography (PET) used to assess brain disorders.

neurology Branch of medicine that studies the organization, function, and treatment of the nervous system.

neuron Nerve cell that sends, receives, and processes information.

neurophysiology Study of the relationship between nervous system structure and function.

neuropsychiatry Medical specialty combining neurology and psychiatry. Emphasizes somatic substructure on which emotions are based and the central nervous system organic neuroreceptors, central nervous system binding sites for neurotransmitters, psychoactive drugs, and hormones.

neurosis An older term for all kinds of emotional disturbances other than psychosis. Neurosis implies subjective psychological discomfort or pain beyond what is appropriate to the conditions of ones life. The disturbance is relatively enduring or recurrent without treatment, not limited to a mild transitory reaction to stress, and has no demonstrable organic etiology.

neurotransmitter Chemical substance released by nerve cell endings in the central nervous system that transmits impulses across synapses between neurons.

norepinephrine Catecholamine neurotransmitter, also called noradrenalin, found in both the peripheral and the central nervous system that helps to regulate arousal, blood pressure, and sleep. Excessive amounts may provoke anxiety.

nyctophobia Fear of night.

obsession Persistent and recurrent idea, thought, impulse, or image that cannot be eliminated by logic or reasoning. An obsession is intrusive, distressing, involuntary, and recognized as being excessive and unreasonable even though it is the product of ones mind.

obsessive-compulsive disorder (OCD) Anxiety disorder characterized by obsessions, compulsions, or both; OCD symptoms are distressing, time-consuming, and significantly interfere with ones normal routine, occupational functioning, usual social activities or relationships with others.

obsessive-compulsive spectrum disorders Conditions that have obsessive-compulsive qualities and similarities to obsessive-compulsive disorder.

ochlophobia Fear of crowds.

odynophobia Fear of pain.

operant conditioning (instrumental conditioning) Process by which the results of a person's behavior determine whether the behavior is more or less likely to occur in the future.

ophidiophobia Fear of snakes.

orientation Awareness of oneself in relation to person, place, and time.

overstimulation Excitation that exceeds the subject's or system's ability to master or discharge it. Since the psyche has a finite capacity for tension, exceeding that capacity with excessive or repeated stimulation constitutes a trauma, and pain (anxiety) is experienced. Anxiety becomes a danger signal and a defense against being overwhelmed.

palpitations Sensation of irregular or rapid beating of the heart. Described as fluttering, throbbing, or pounding.

panic Acute, intense, overwhelming anxiety producing feelings of impending doom and physiological changes.

panic attack Period of intense fear or discomfort with the abrupt development of physical symptoms and fear of dying, going crazy, or losing control, reaching a peak within 10 minutes. Symptoms may include dizziness, faintness, trembling or shaking, sweating, choking, shortness of breath or smothering sensations, nausea or abdominal distress, flushes or chills, chest pain or discomfort, rapid heart rate, and palpitations.

panic disorder Recurrent, unexpected panic attacks, at least one of which is followed by a month or more of persistent concern about having another attack. There are two types: with or without agoraphobia.

panphobia Fear of everything.

parasympathetic nervous system Part of the autonomic nervous system that controls the life-sustaining organs under normal, danger-free conditions.

paresthesia Abnormal spontaneous tactile sensations, often described as tingling, creeping, tickling, prickling, or burning.

pathognomic Indicative of a disease or illness, especially characteristic symptoms.

pedophobia Fear of children.

performance anxiety Form of social anxiety in which excessive fear relates to performing a specific task in front of others.

pharmacodynamics Study of the biochemical and physiological effects of drugs and their mechanisms of action.

pharmacokinetics Study of the process amd rates of drug absorption, distribution, metabolism, and disposition in the organism.

pharmacotherapy Treatment of disease through the use of pharmaceutical medications.

phobia Intense, persistent, pathological, unrealistic, fear of an object or situation, which the subject recognizes as excessive or unreasonable, but cannot dispel it. The phobic stimulus is avoided or endured with marked distress.

phonophobia Fear of or increased sensitivity to loud noises.

photophobia Fear of light or sensitivity to light.

placebo Treatment condition used to control for the placebo effect where the treatment has no real effect of its own.

poinephobia Fear of punishment.

posttraumatic stress disorder (PTSD) Anxiety disorder in which exposure to an exceptional mental or physical stressor is followed by avoidance, numbing sensation, persistent reexperiencing of the event, and increased arousal, sometimes occurring immediately and sometimes not until 6 months or more after the stress. The trauma typically includes witnessing, experiencing, or confronting an event that involves actual or threatened death or injury, or a threat to the physical integrity of oneself or others. Reactions include helplessness, fear and horror.

pnigerophobia Fear of smothering.

prevalence Total number of cases that exist within a unit of population.

psyche The mind.

psychiatry The medical science that deals with the origin, prevention, diagnosis, and treatment of mental disorders.

psychic trauma An intrapsychic event brought on by exposure to an unanticipated danger.

psychology A profession, an academic discipline, and a science dealing with the study of mental processes and behavior.

psychomotor Referring to combined physical and mental activity.

psychomotor agitation Excessive motor activity associated with a feeling of inner tension. Usually nonproductive and repetitious and consists of behavior such as inability to sit still, pacing, and wringing of hands.

psychopharmacology The study of the effects of psychoactive substances on behavior. Clinical psychopharmacology more specifically includes both the study of drug effects in patients and the expert use of drugs in the treatment of psychiatric conditions.

psychotherapy Form of therapy in which a person relieves symptoms or resolves problems through verbal interaction. Talk therapy.

psychotropic Drug that has a special effect on the psyche.

pyrophobia Fear of fire.

rebound Return of original symptoms when treatment stops.

receptor Specialized area on a nerve membrane, blood vessel, or muscle that receives the chemical stimulation that activates or inhibits.

relapse Return of symptoms associated with the present episode of illness after the symptoms had been reduced or eliminated for a brief period.

relaxation training Use of relaxation techniques to help control the physical and mental state in the treatment of mental disorders.

remission Abatement of an illness.

response prevention Theraputic technique where stimuli are presented but the individual is not permitted to respond with the typical response.

ritual Formalized, repetitive activity to reduce anxiety.

rumination Constant preoccupation with thinking about a single theme or idea.

scholionophobia Fear of school.

sciophobia Fear of shadows.

selective serotonin reuptake inhibitors (SSRIs) Class of antidepressants that increase the amount of serotonin available at the synapse, used to treat major depression, many of the anxiety disorders, and other psychiatric disorders. Also sometimes referred to as serotonin reuptake inhibitors (SRIs).

sensorium That portion of the brain that functions as a center of sensations.

serotonin Central nervous system neurotransmitter involved in mood, sleep, appetite, sexual drive, impulsive and aggressive behavior. When decreased or deficient, may lead to various problems including anxiety disorders and depression.

serotonin-norepinephrine reuptake inhibitors (SNRIs) Class of antidepressants used for the treatment of anxiety disorders, depression, as well as other disorders.

serotonin receptor Protein that binds the neurotransmitter serotonin, becomes activated, and then activates serotonin neurons and pathways.

serotonin syndrome Excessive stimulation of serotonin receptors. Symptoms include mental confusion, lethargy, flushing, diaphoresis, tremor, hyperthermia, hypertonicity, renal failure, and death.

social phobia (social anxiety disorder) Intense anxiety of being judged by others in social situations.

specific phobia (also known as **single, simple phobia**) Real, intense, but illogical fear of a specific animal, object, situation or activity.

stress Physical and psychological result of internal or external pressure.

substrate Drug or substance metabolized by an enzyme.

sympathetic nervous system Part of the autonomic nervous system that responds to dangerous or threatening situations by preparing a person physiologically for fight or flight. Plays a role in the body's homeostasis.

synapse Gap between one nerve cell membrane and another, through which the nerve impulse is passed chemically or electrically.

syndrome Configuration of symptoms that occur together and constitute a recognizable condition.

systematic desensitization Behavior therapy procedure widely used to modify behaviors.

tension Physiological or psychic uneasiness, arousal, or pressure toward action.

terminal insomnia Early morning awakening or waking up at least 2 hours before planning to wake up.

theophobia Fear of God.

topophobia Fear of stage fright.

transference Intense feelings directed toward the therapist that many individuals experience in the process of therapy.

tranquilizer Medication that decreases anxiety and agitation.

tricyclic antidepressants Older class of antidepressants that enhance the concentration of central nervous system norepinephrine and serotonin, useful in some anxiety disorders, depression, and other disorders.

triskaidekaphobia Fear of the number thirteen.

tropophobia Fear of moving or making changes.

References

1. Shahrokh NC, Hales RE, ed. American Psychiatric Glossary, 8th ed. Arlington, VA: American Psychiatric Publishing, Inc. 2003.
2. http://www.adaa.org/gettinghelp/glossary.asp.
3. Foa EB, Andrews LW. If Your Adolescent Has an Anxiety Disorder. New York: Oxford University Press, 2006:203–209.
4. Othmer E, Othmer S, Othmer JP. Diagnosis and psychiatry: examination of the psychiatric patient. In: Sadock BJ, Sadock VA, eds. Kaplan and Sadock's Comprehensive Textbook of Psychiatry, 8th ed., vol.1. Philadelphia: Lippincott Williams and Wilkins, 2005: 849–859.
5. Yager J, Giltin MJ. Clinical manifestations of psychiatric disorders. In: Sadock BJ, Sadock VA, eds. Kaplan and Sadock Sadock's Comprehensive Textbook of Psychiatry, 8th ed., vol.1. Philadelphia: Lippincott Williams and Wilkins, 2005:993.
6. http://allpsych.com/dictionary.
7. Venes D, ed. Taber's Cyclopedic Medical Dictionary, 20th ed. Philadelphia: F.A. Davis Company, 2005.

Index